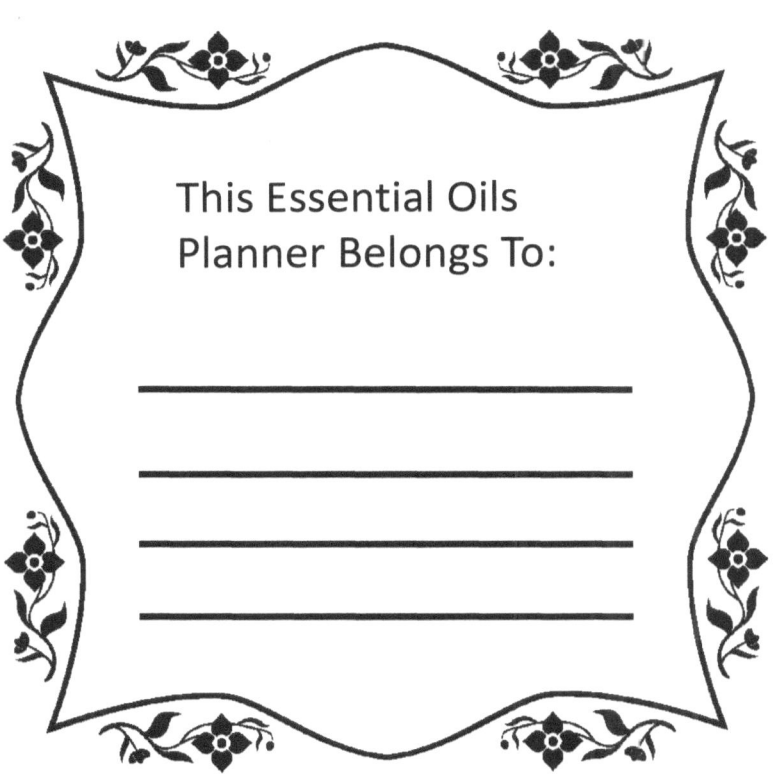

This Essential Oils
Planner Belongs To:

_____

_____

_____

_____

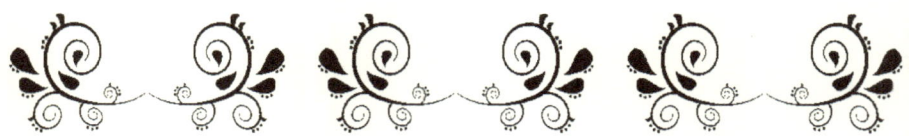

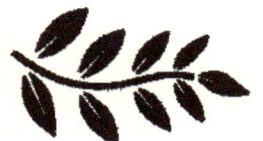

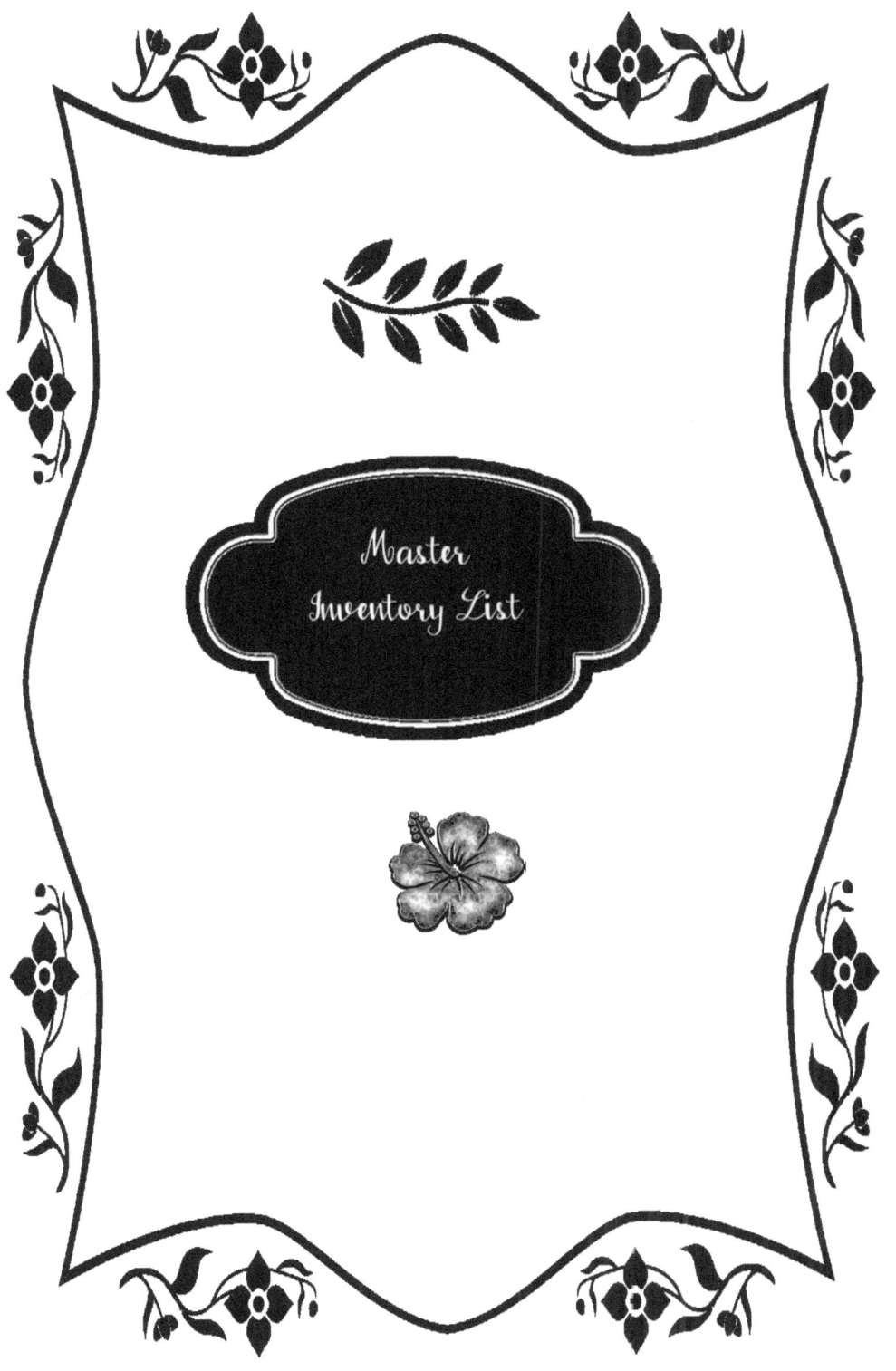

Master
Inventory List

Master Inventory List

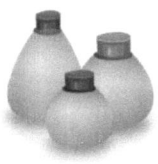

Oil Name	Uses	Date of Purchase

Master Inventory List

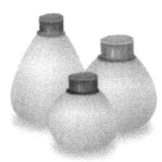

Oil Name	Uses	Date of Purchase

Master Inventory List

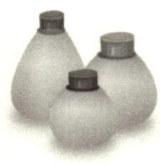

Oil Name	Uses	Date of Purchase

Master Inventory List

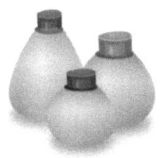

Oil Name	Uses	Date of Purchase

Master Inventory List

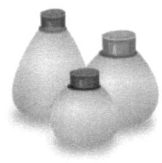

Oil Name	Uses	Date of Purchase

Master Inventory List

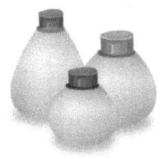

Oil Name	Uses	Date of Purchase

Master Inventory List

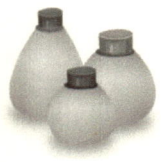

Oil Name	Uses	Date of Purchase

Master Inventory List

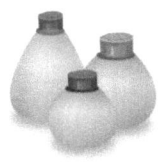

Oil Name	Uses	Date of Purchase

Master Inventory List

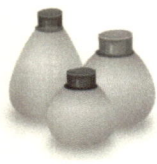

Oil Name	Uses	Date of Purchase

Master Inventory List

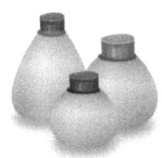

Oil Name	Uses	Date of Purchase

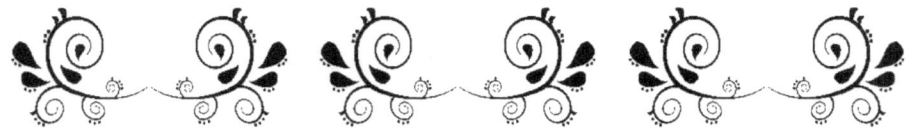

Treatment Journal

Date	What Was Used	Ailment	Application	Result

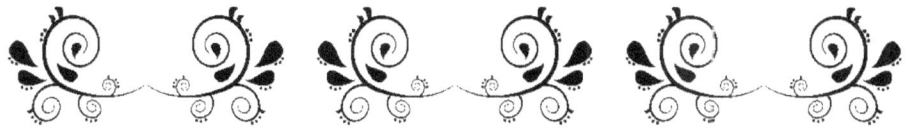

Treatment Journal

Date	What Was Used	Ailment	Application	Result

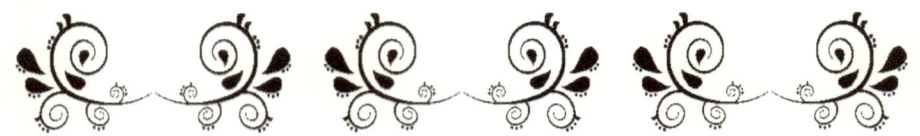

Treatment Journal

Date	What Was Used	Ailment	Application	Result

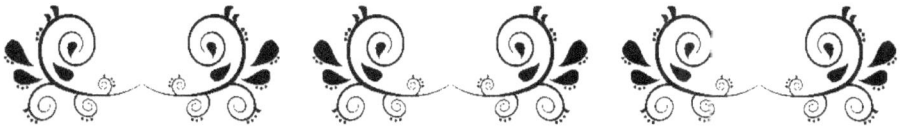

Treatment Journal

Date	What Was Used	Ailment	Application	Result

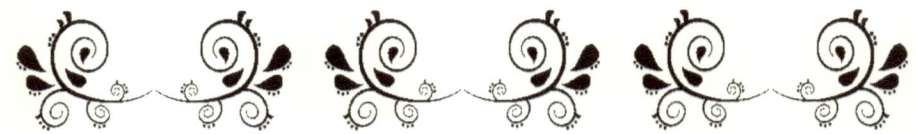

Treatment Journal

Date	What Was Used	Ailment	Application	Result

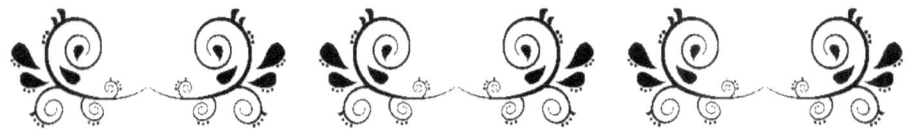

Treatment Journal

Date	What Was Used	Ailment	Application	Result

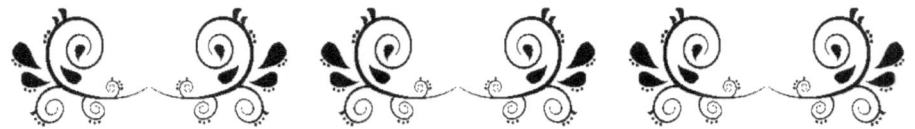

Treatment Journal

Date	What Was Used	Ailment	Application	Result

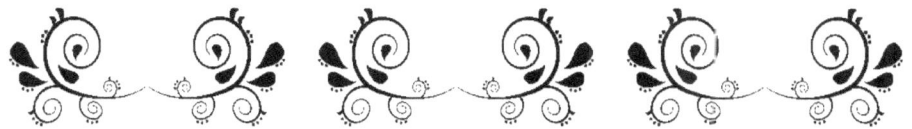

Treatment Journal

Date	What Was Used	Ailment	Application	Result

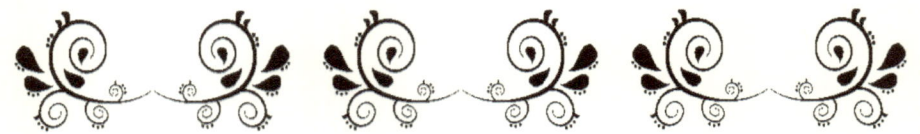

Treatment Journal

Date	What Was Used	Ailment	Application	Result

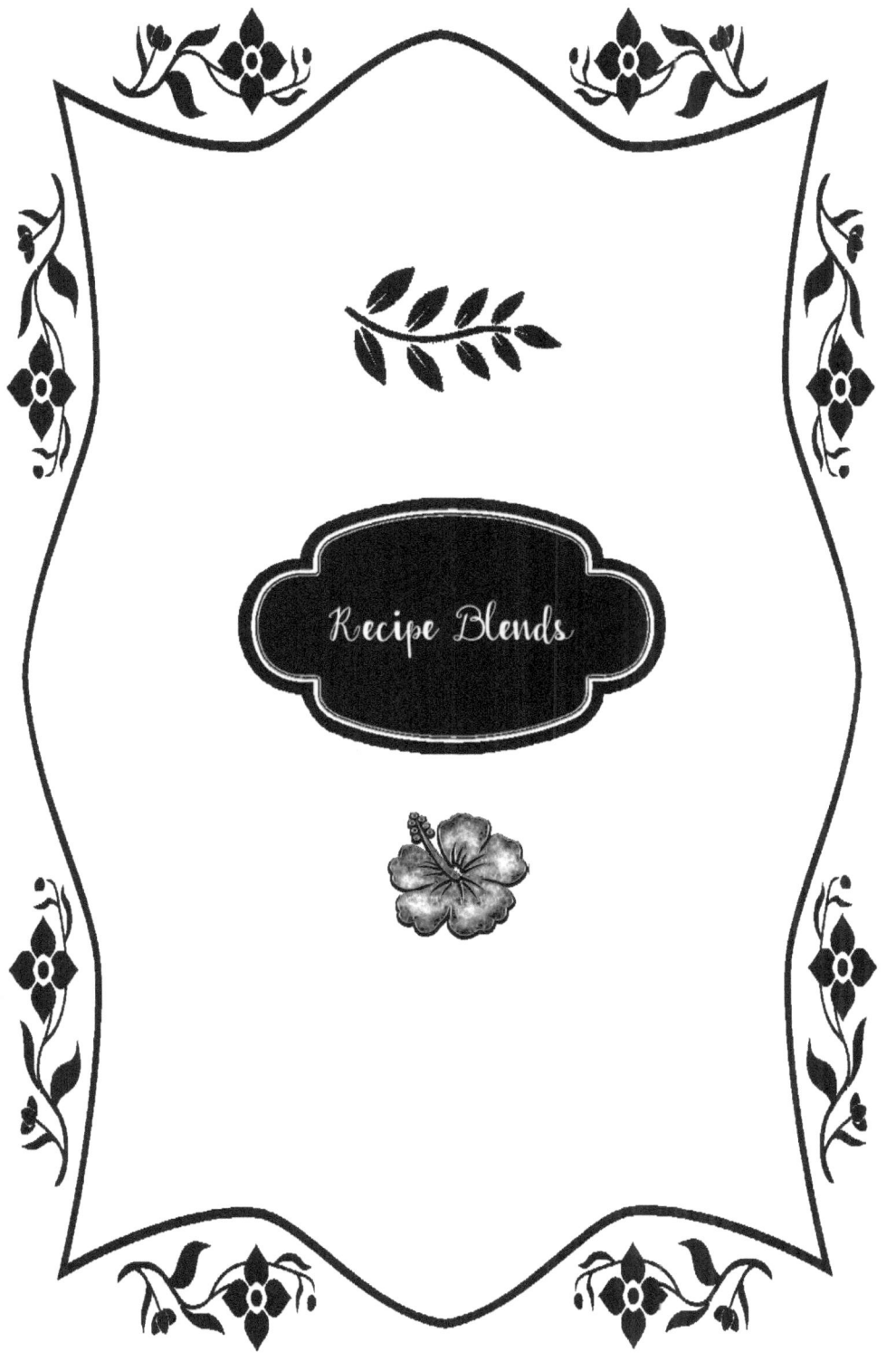

Recipe Blends

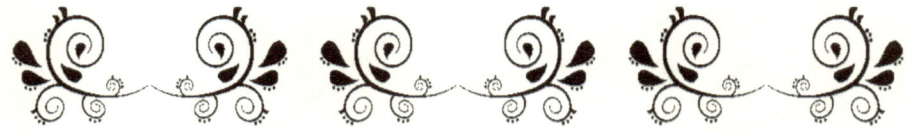

Recipe Index

Recipe	Page

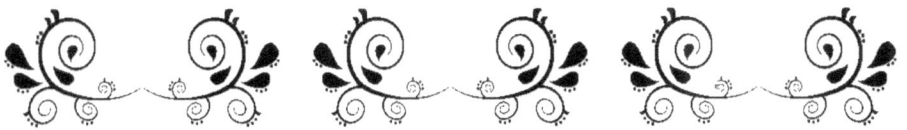

Recipe Index

Recipe	Page

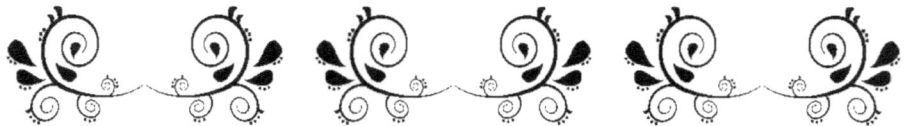

Recipe Index

Recipe	Page

Recipe Blend

_____

_____

_____

_____

_____

_____

Recipe Blend

_____

_____

_____

_____

_____

_____

Recipe Blend

_____

_____

_____

_____

_____

_____

Recipe Blend

_____

_____

_____

_____

_____

_____

Recipe Blend

_____

_____

_____

_____

_____

_____

Recipe Blend

_____

_____

_____

_____

_____

_____

Recipe Blend

_____

_____

_____

_____

_____

_____

Recipe Blend

_____

_____

_____

_____

_____

_____

Recipe Blend

_____

_____

_____

_____

_____

_____

Recipe Blend

_____

_____

_____

_____

_____

_____

Recipe Blend

_____

_____

_____

_____

_____

_____

Recipe Blend

_____

_____

_____

_____

_____

_____

Recipe Blend

_____

_____

_____

_____

_____

_____

Recipe Blend

_____

_____

_____

_____

_____

_____

Recipe Blend

_____

_____

_____

_____

_____

_____

Recipe Blend

_____

_____

_____

_____

_____

_____

Recipe Blend

_____

_____

_____

_____

_____

_____

Recipe Blend

_____

_____

_____

_____

_____

_____

Recipe Blend

_____

_____

_____

_____

_____

_____

Recipe Blend

_____

_____

_____

_____

_____

_____

Recipe Blend

Recipe Blend

Recipe Blend

_____

_____

_____

_____

_____

_____

Recipe Blend

_____

_____

_____

_____

_____

_____

Recipe Blend

_____

_____

_____

_____

_____

_____

Recipe Blend

_____

_____

_____

_____

_____

_____

Recipe Blend

Recipe Blend

Recipe Blend

_____

_____

_____

_____

_____

_____

Recipe Blend

_____

_____

_____

_____

_____

_____

Recipe Blend

_____

_____

_____

_____

_____

_____

Recipe Blend

_____

_____

_____

_____

_____

_____

Recipe Blend

_____

_____

_____

_____

_____

_____

Recipe Blend

_____

_____

_____

_____

_____

_____

Recipe Blend

_____

_____

_____

_____

_____

_____

Recipe Blend

_____

_____

_____

_____

_____

_____

Recipe Blend

_____

_____

_____

_____

_____

_____

Recipe Blend

_____

_____

_____

_____

_____

_____

Recipe Blend

Recipe Blend

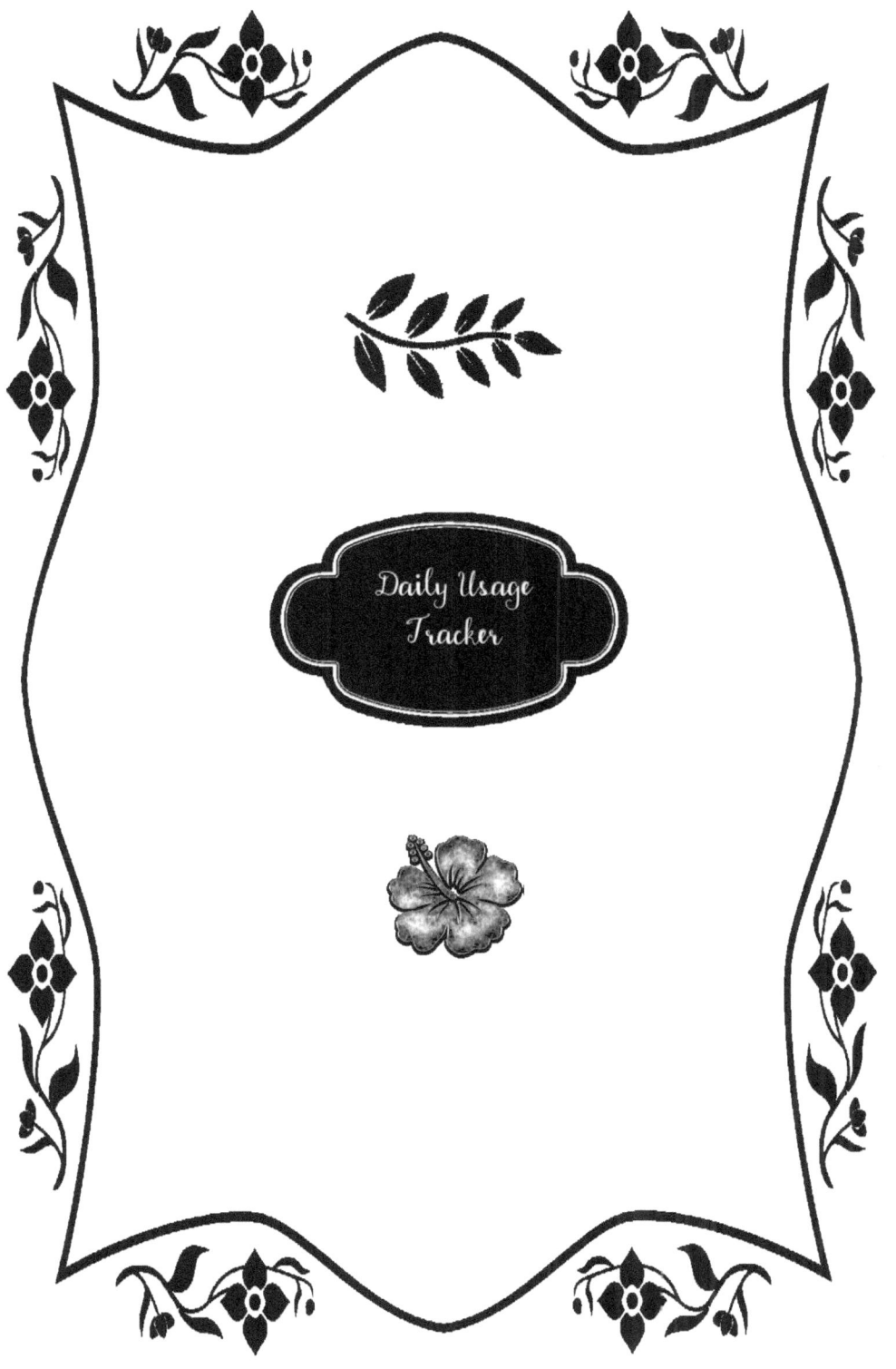

Daily Usage
Tracker

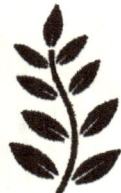

Daily Oil Usage Tracker

Date: _____

	S	M	T	W	T	F	S
Lavender							
Bergamot							
Eucalyptus							
Frankincense							
Lemon							

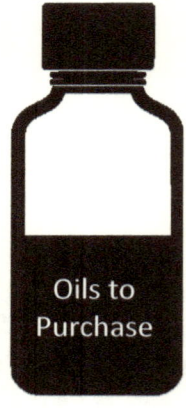

Oils to Purchase

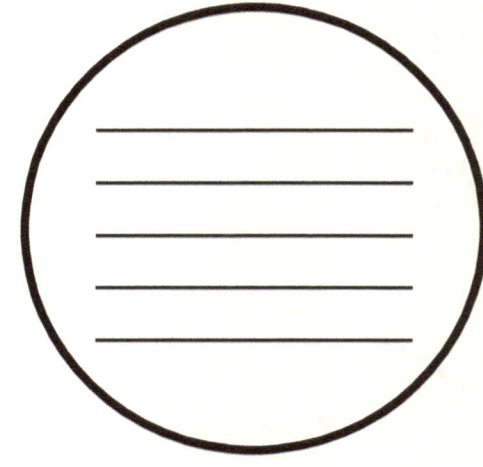

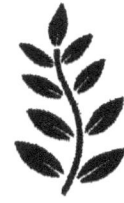

Daily Oil Usage Tracker

Date: _____

	S	M	T	W	T	F	S
Lavender							
Bergamot							
Eucalyptus							
Frankincense							
Lemon							

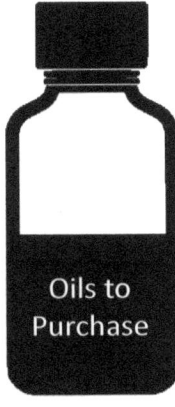

Oils to Purchase

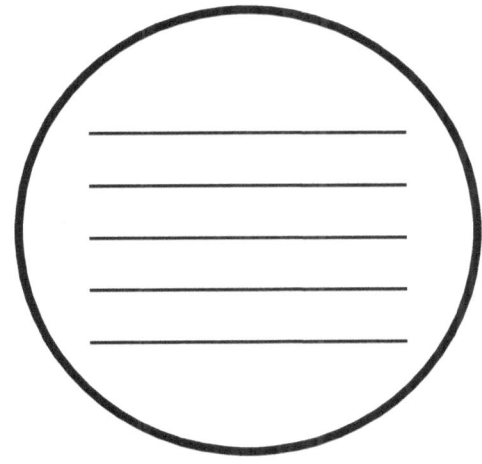

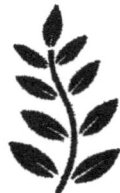

Daily Oil Usage Tracker

Date: _____

	S	M	T	W	T	F	S
Lavender							
Bergamot							
Eucalyptus							
Frankincense							
Lemon							

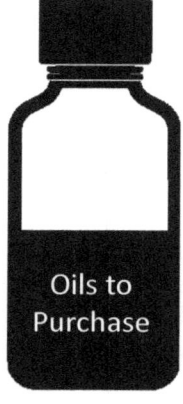

Oils to Purchase

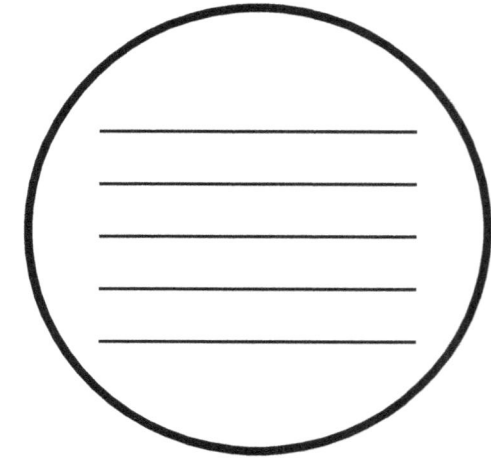

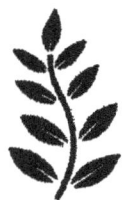

Daily Oil Usage Tracker

Date: _____

	S	M	T	W	T	F	S
Lavender							
Bergamot							
Eucalyptus							
Frankincense							
Lemon							

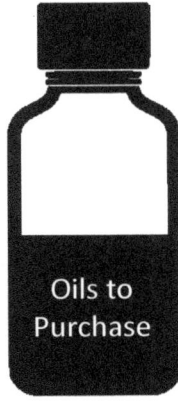

Oils to Purchase

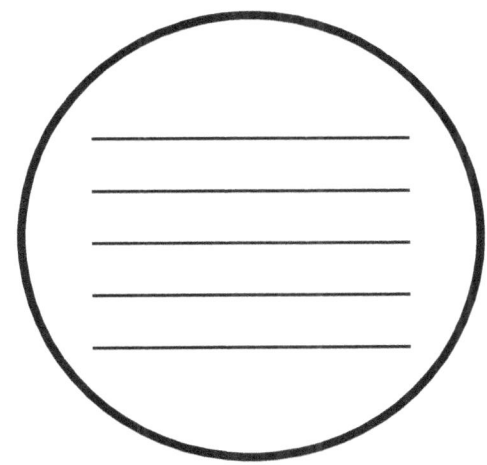

Daily Oil Usage Tracker

Date: _____

	S	M	T	W	T	F	S
Lavender							
Bergamot							
Eucalyptus							
Frankincense							
Lemon							

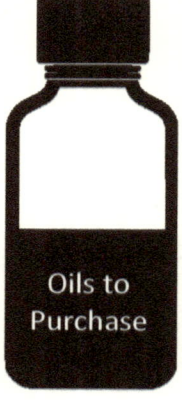

Oils to Purchase

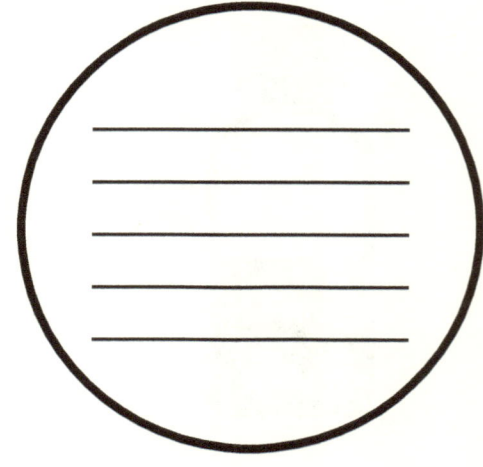

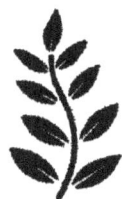

Daily Oil Usage Tracker

Date: _____

	S	M	T	W	T	F	S
Lavender							
Bergamot							
Eucalyptus							
Frankincense							
Lemon							

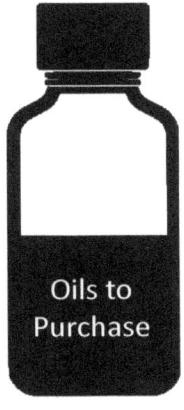

Oils to Purchase

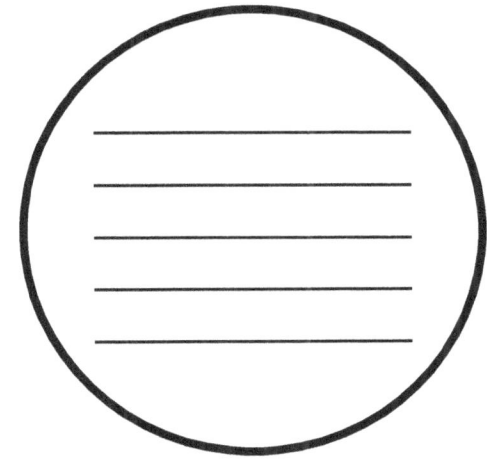

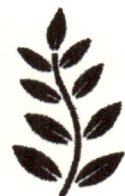

Daily Oil Usage Tracker

Date: _____

	S	M	T	W	T	F	S
Lavender							
Bergamot							
Eucalyptus							
Frankincense							
Lemon							

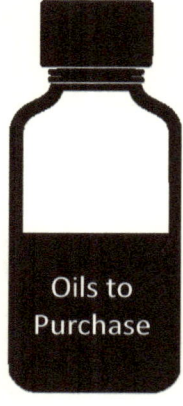

Oils to Purchase

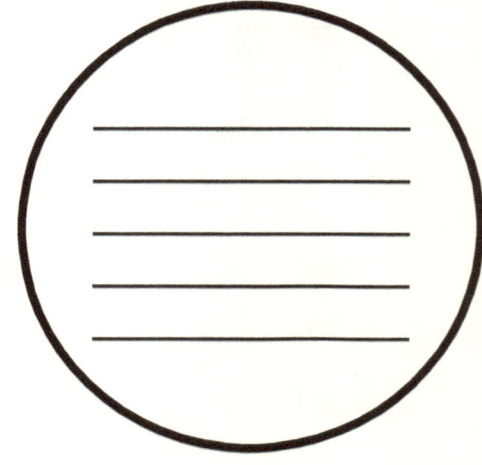

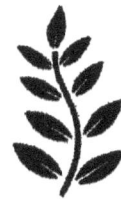

Daily Oil Usage Tracker

Date: _____

	S	M	T	W	T	F	S
Lavender							
Bergamot							
Eucalyptus							
Frankincense							
Lemon							

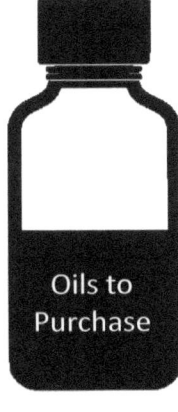

Oils to Purchase

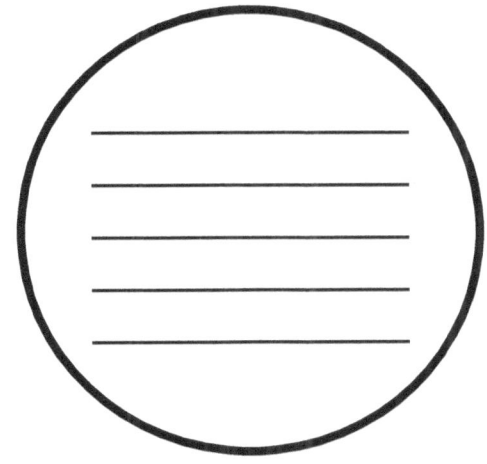

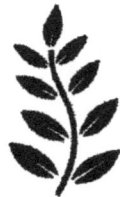

Daily Oil Usage Tracker

Date: _____

	S	M	T	W	T	F	S
Lavender							
Bergamot							
Eucalyptus							
Frankincense							
Lemon							

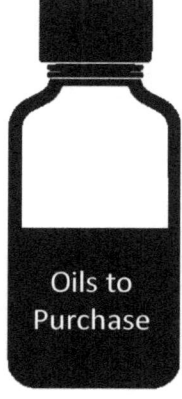

Oils to Purchase

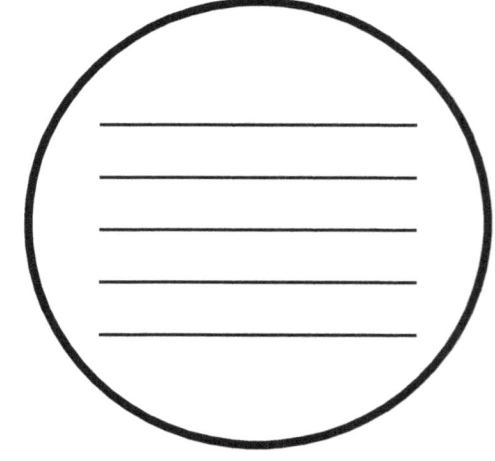

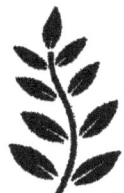

Daily Oil Usage Tracker

Date: _____

	S	M	T	W	T	F	S
Lavender							
Bergamot							
Eucalyptus							
Frankincense							
Lemon							

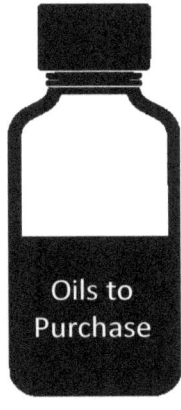

Oils to Purchase

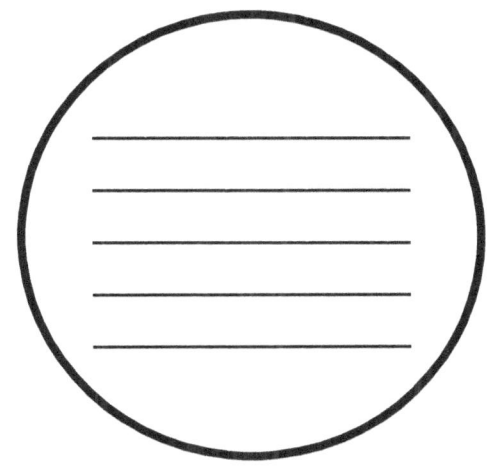

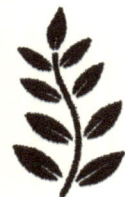

Daily Oil Usage Tracker

Date: _____

	S	M	T	W	T	F	S
Lavender							
Bergamot							
Eucalyptus							
Frankincense							
Lemon							

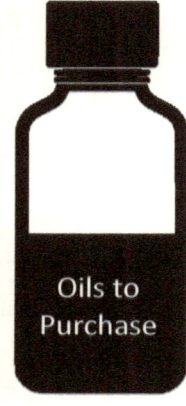

Oils to Purchase

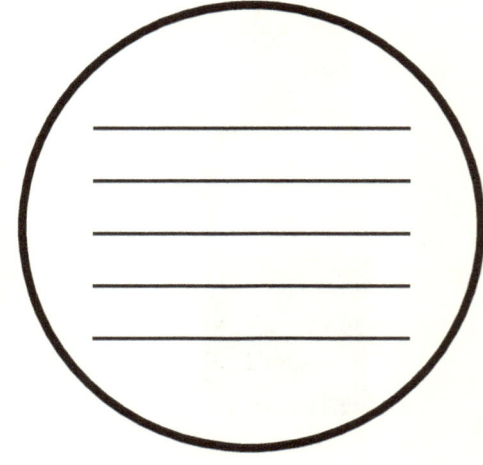

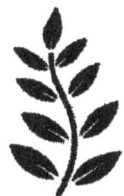

Daily Oil Usage Tracker

Date: _____

	S	M	T	W	T	F	S
Lavender							
Bergamot							
Eucalyptus							
Frankincense							
Lemon							

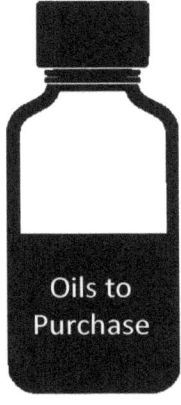

Oils to Purchase

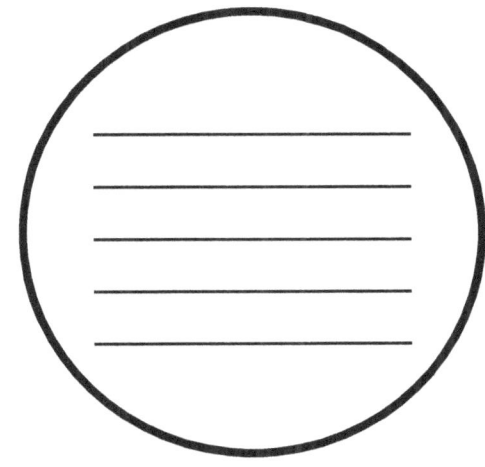

Daily Oil Usage Tracker

Date: _____

	S	M	T	W	T	F	S
Lavender							
Bergamot							
Eucalyptus							
Frankincense							
Lemon							

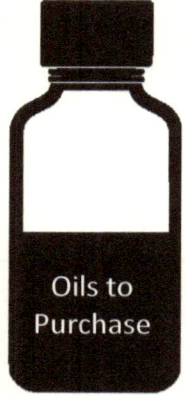

Oils to Purchase

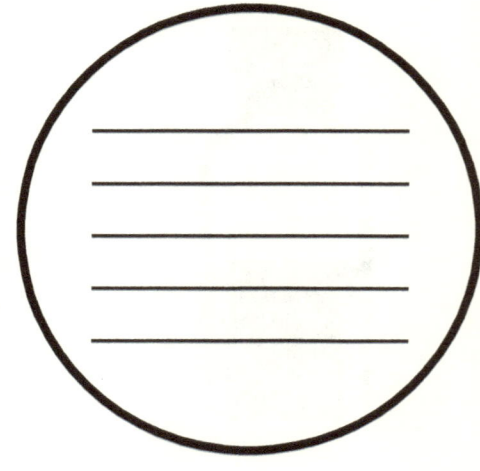

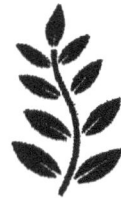

Daily Oil Usage Tracker

Date: _____

	S	M	T	W	T	F	S
Lavender							
Bergamot							
Eucalyptus							
Frankincense							
Lemon							

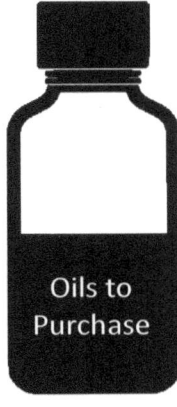

Oils to Purchase

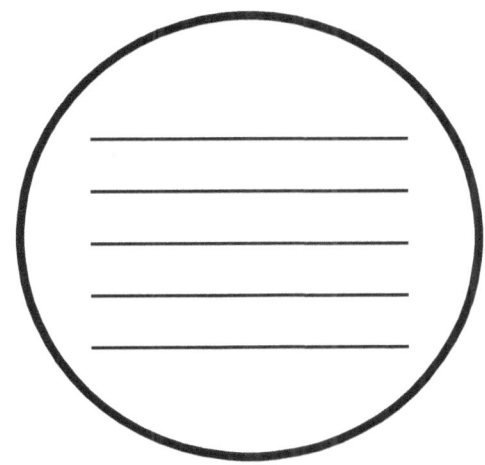

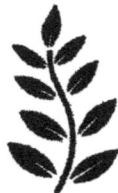

Daily Oil Usage Tracker

Date: _____

	S	M	T	W	T	F	S
Lavender							
Bergamot							
Eucalyptus							
Frankincense							
Lemon							

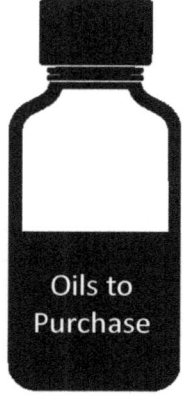

Oils to Purchase

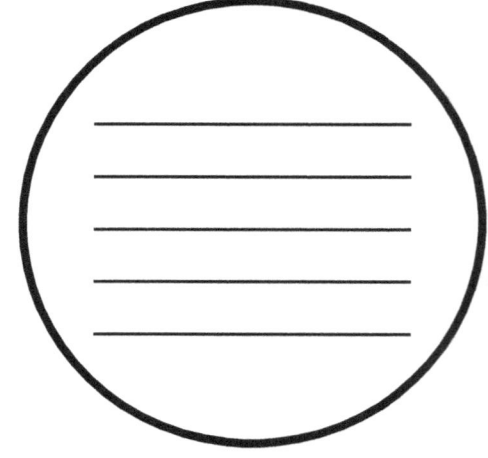

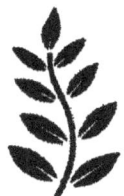

Daily Oil Usage Tracker

Date: _____

	S	M	T	W	T	F	S
Lavender							
Bergamot							
Eucalyptus							
Frankincense							
Lemon							

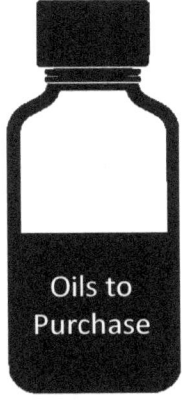

Oils to Purchase

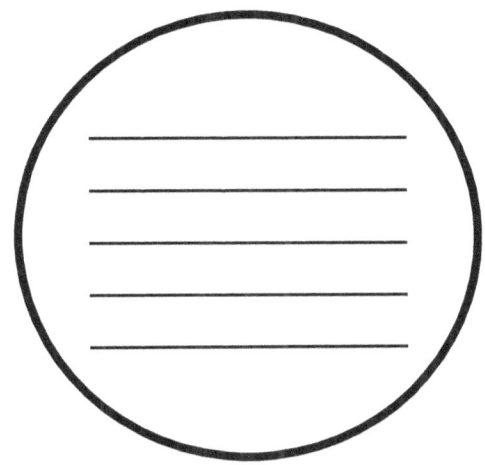

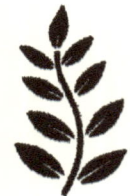

Daily Oil Usage Tracker

Date: _____

	S	M	T	W	T	F	S
Lavender							
Bergamot							
Eucalyptus							
Frankincense							
Lemon							

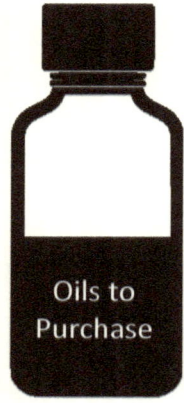

Oils to Purchase

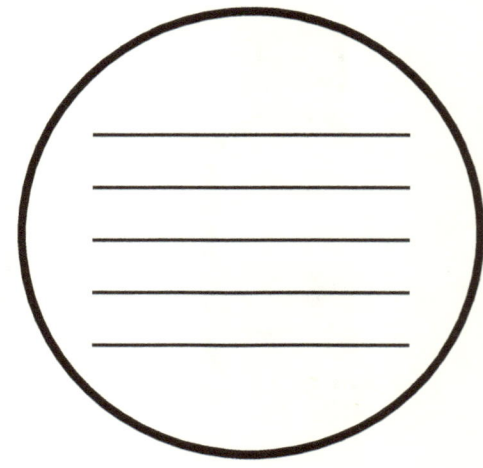

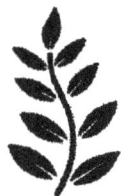

Daily Oil Usage Tracker

Date: _____

	S	M	T	W	T	F	S
Lavender							
Bergamot							
Eucalyptus							
Frankincense							
Lemon							

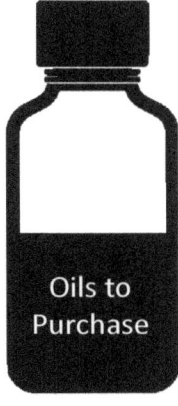

Oils to Purchase

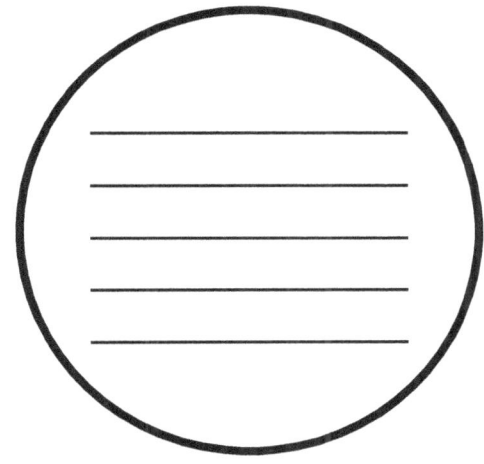

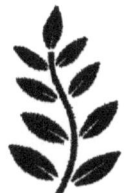

Daily Oil Usage Tracker

Date: _____

	S	M	T	W	T	F	S
Lavender							
Bergamot							
Eucalyptus							
Frankincense							
Lemon							

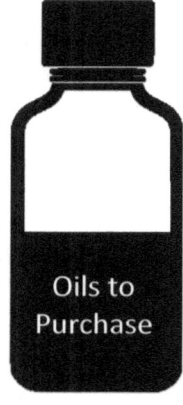

Oils to Purchase

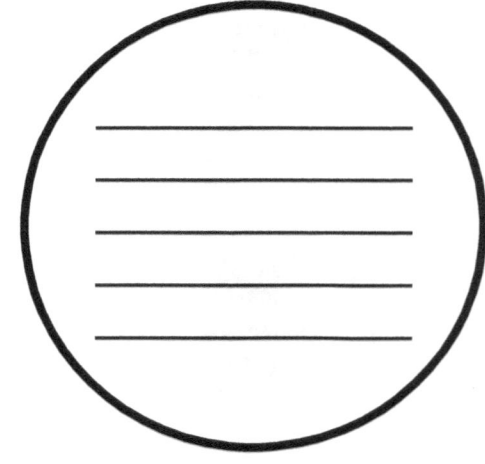

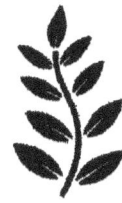

Daily Oil Usage Tracker

Date: _____

	S	M	T	W	T	F	S
Lavender							
Bergamot							
Eucalyptus							
Frankincense							
Lemon							

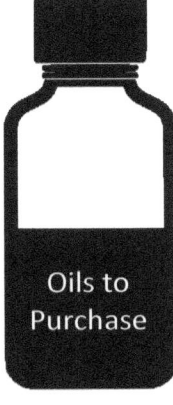

Oils to Purchase

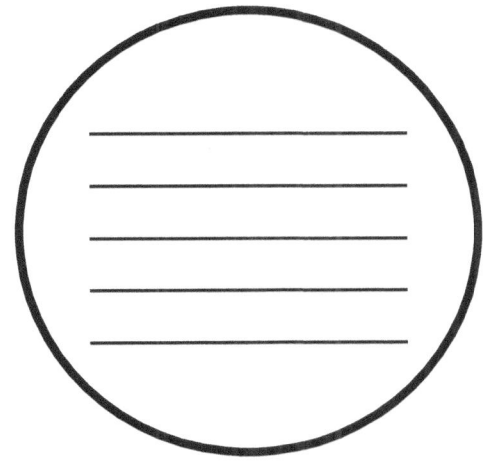

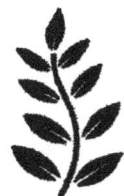

Daily Oil Usage Tracker

Date: _____

	S	M	T	W	T	F	S
Lavender							
Bergamot							
Eucalyptus							
Frankincense							
Lemon							

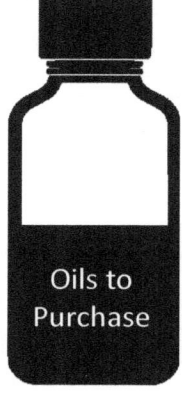

Oils to Purchase

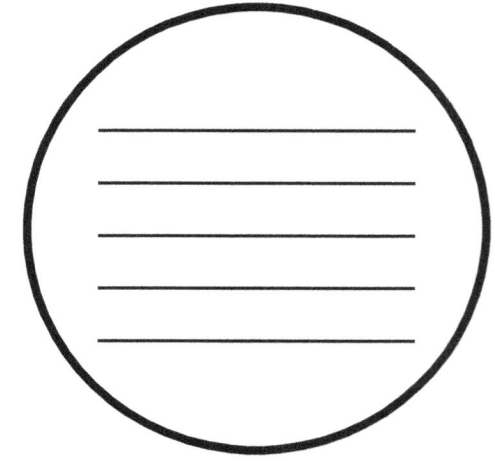

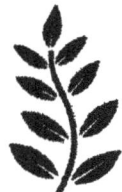

Daily Oil Usage Tracker

Date: _____

	S	M	T	W	T	F	S
Lavender							
Bergamot							
Eucalyptus							
Frankincense							
Lemon							

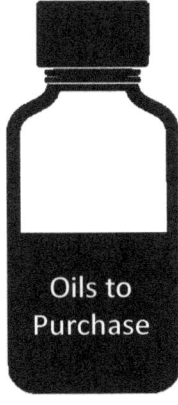

Oils to Purchase

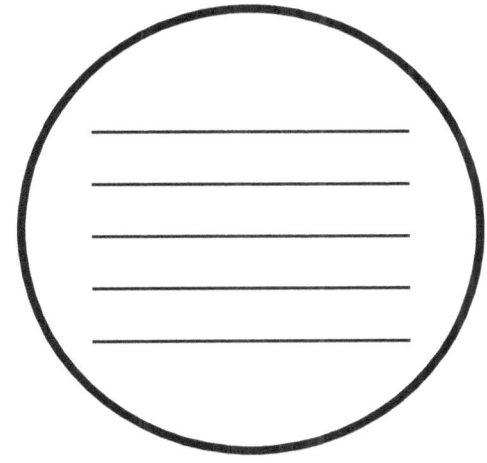

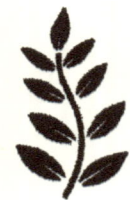

Daily Oil Usage Tracker

Date: _____

	S	M	T	W	T	F	S
Lavender							
Bergamot							
Eucalyptus							
Frankincense							
Lemon							

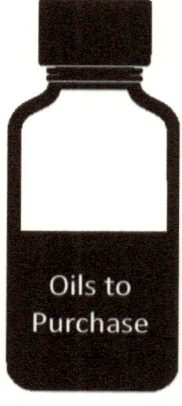

Oils to Purchase

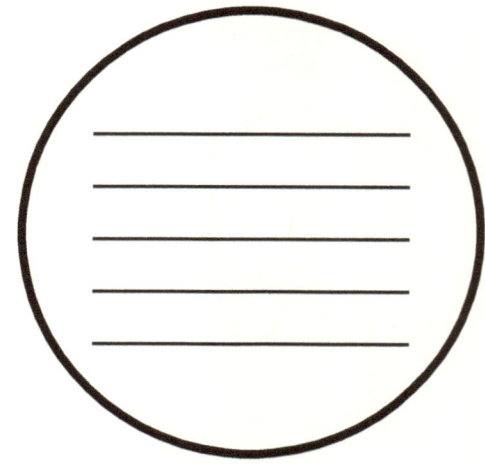

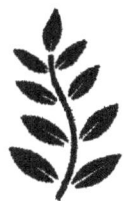

Daily Oil Usage Tracker

Date: _____

	S	M	T	W	T	F	S
Lavender							
Bergamot							
Eucalyptus							
Frankincense							
Lemon							

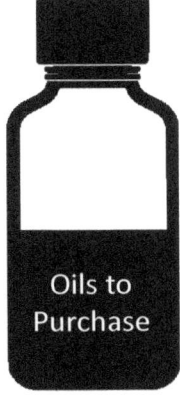

Oils to Purchase

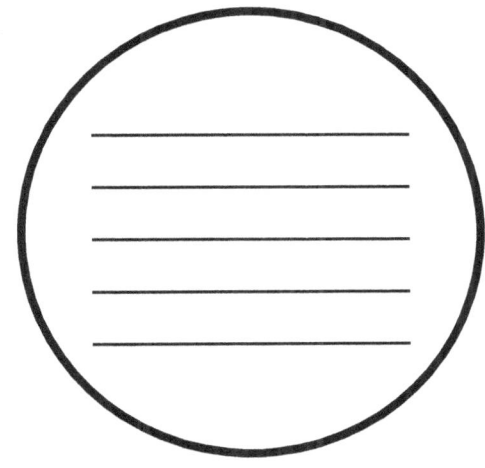

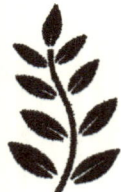

Daily Oil Usage Tracker

Date: _____

	S	M	T	W	T	F	S
Lavender							
Bergamot							
Eucalyptus							
Frankincense							
Lemon							

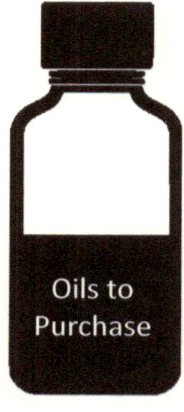

Oils to Purchase

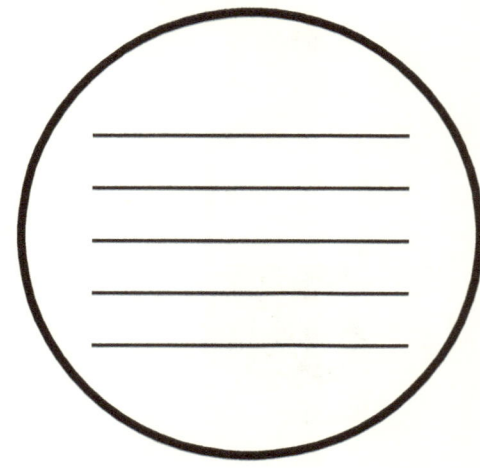

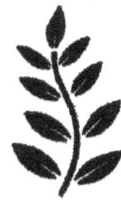

Daily Oil Usage Tracker

Date: _____

	S	M	T	W	T	F	S
Lavender							
Bergamot							
Eucalyptus							
Frankincense							
Lemon							

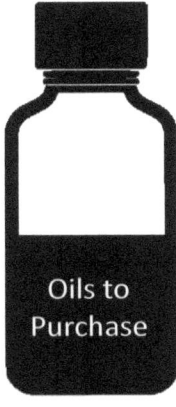

Oils to Purchase

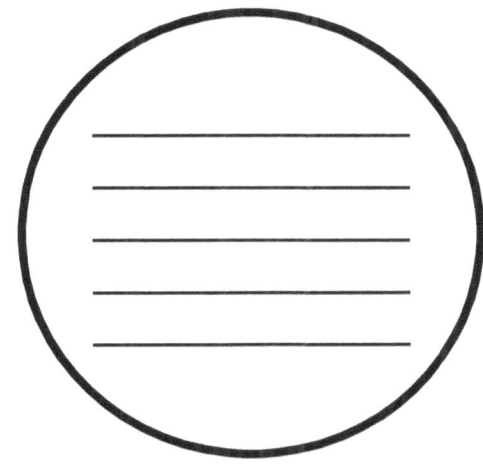

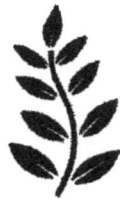

Daily Oil Usage Tracker

Date: _____

	S	M	T	W	T	F	S
Lavender							
Bergamot							
Eucalyptus							
Frankincense							
Lemon							

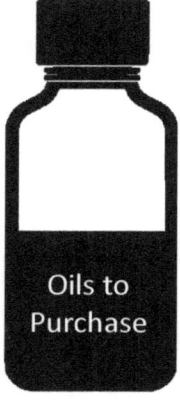

Oils to Purchase

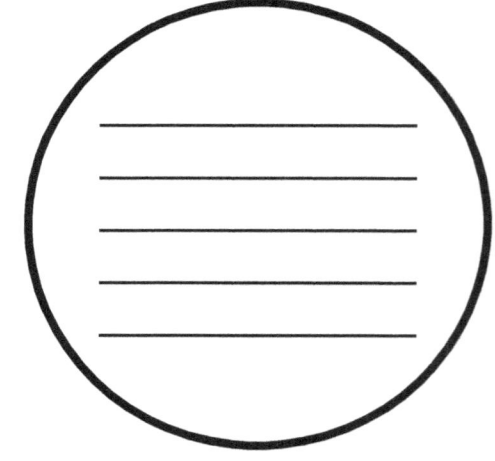

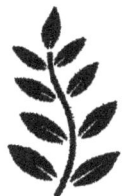

Daily Oil Usage Tracker

Date: _____

	S	M	T	W	T	F	S
Lavender							
Bergamot							
Eucalyptus							
Frankincense							
Lemon							

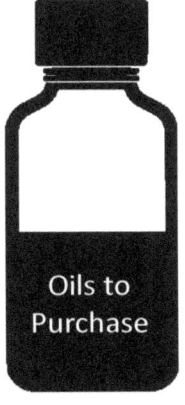

Oils to Purchase

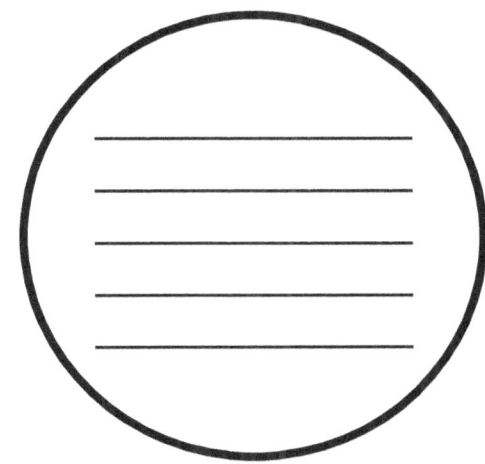

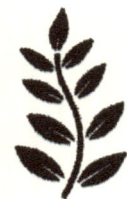

Daily Oil Usage Tracker

Date: _____

	S	M	T	W	T	F	S
Lavender							
Bergamot							
Eucalyptus							
Frankincense							
Lemon							

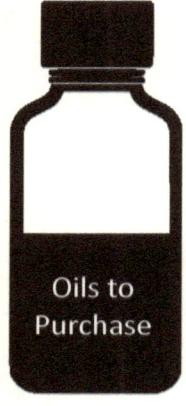

Oils to Purchase

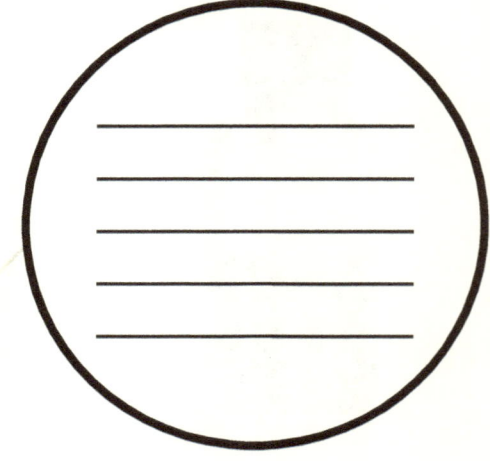

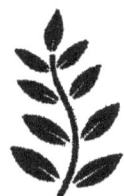

Daily Oil Usage Tracker

Date: _____

	S	M	T	W	T	F	S
Lavender							
Bergamot							
Eucalyptus							
Frankincense							
Lemon							

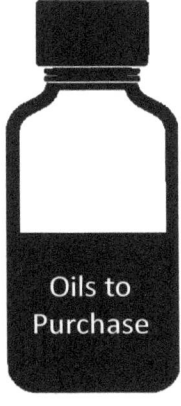

Oils to Purchase

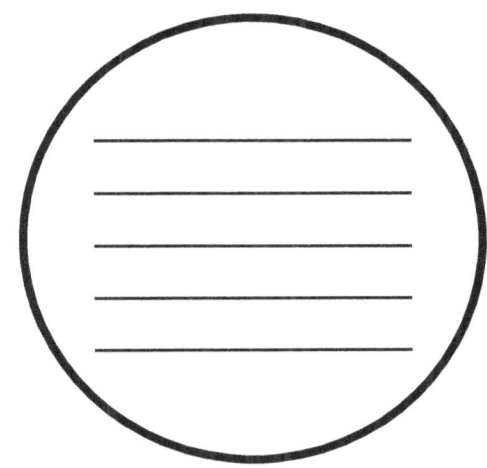

Daily Oil Usage Tracker

Date: _____

	S	M	T	W	T	F	S
Lavender							
Bergamot							
Eucalyptus							
Frankincense							
Lemon							

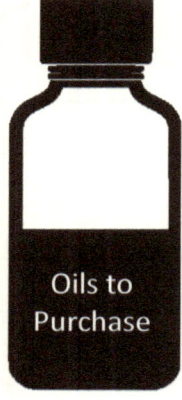

Oils to Purchase

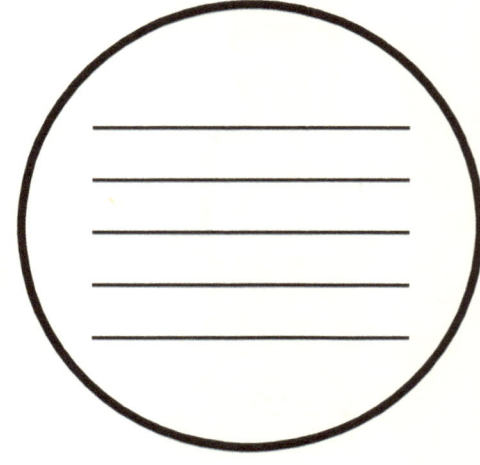

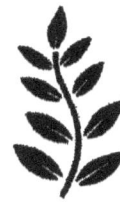

Daily Oil Usage Tracker

Date: _____

	S	M	T	W	T	F	S
Lavender							
Bergamot							
Eucalyptus							
Frankincense							
Lemon							

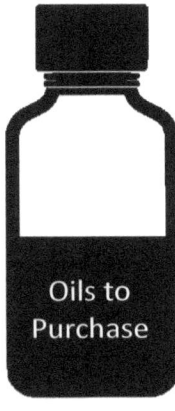

Oils to Purchase

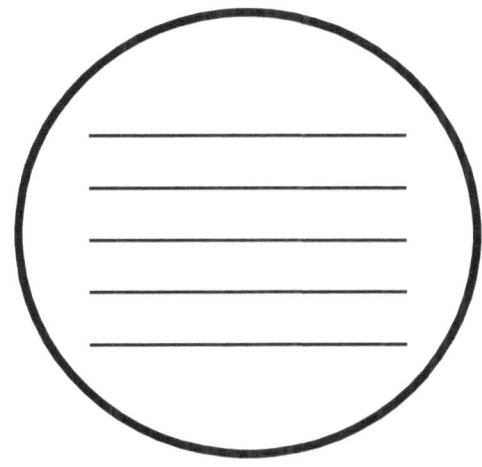

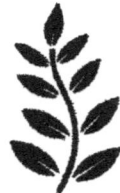

Daily Oil Usage Tracker

Date: _____

	S	M	T	W	T	F	S
Lavender							
Bergamot							
Eucalyptus							
Frankincense							
Lemon							

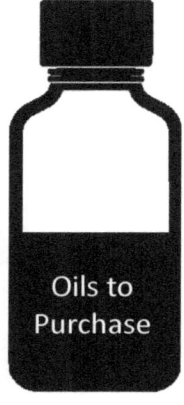

Oils to Purchase

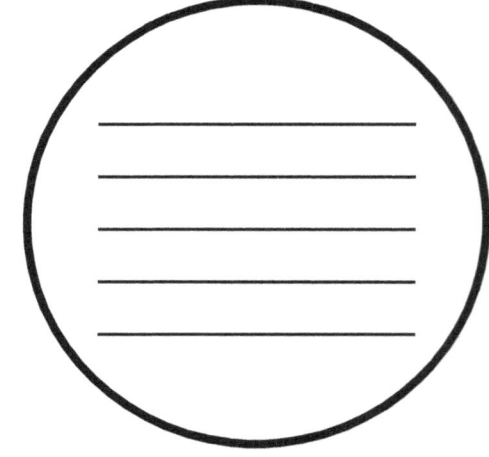

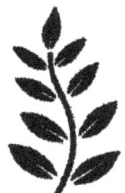

Daily Oil Usage Tracker

Date: _____

	S	M	T	W	T	F	S
Lavender							
Bergamot							
Eucalyptus							
Frankincense							
Lemon							

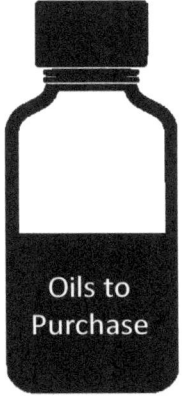

Oils to Purchase

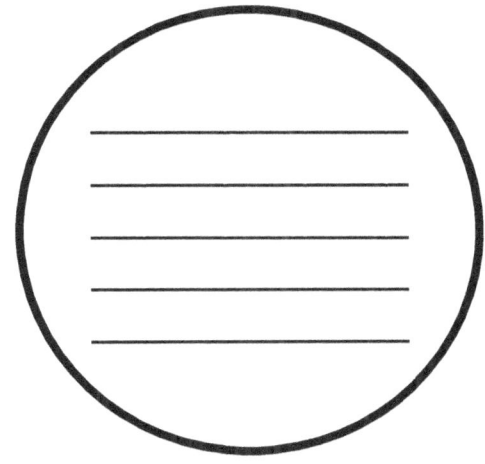

Daily Oil Usage Tracker

Date: _____

	S	M	T	W	T	F	S
Lavender							
Bergamot							
Eucalyptus							
Frankincense							
Lemon							

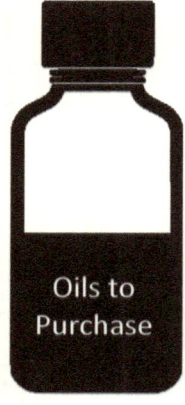

Oils to Purchase

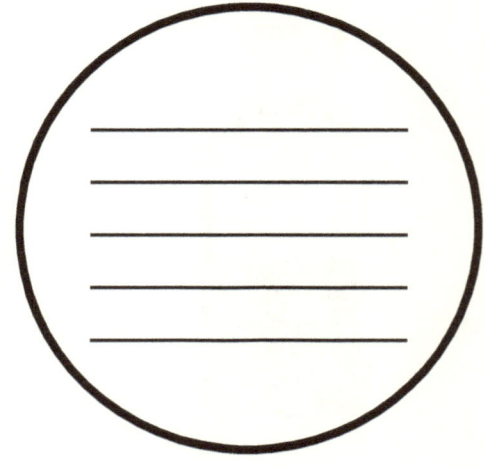

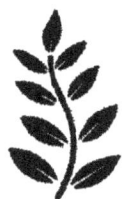

Daily Oil Usage Tracker

Date: _____

	S	M	T	W	T	F	S
Lavender							
Bergamot							
Eucalyptus							
Frankincense							
Lemon							

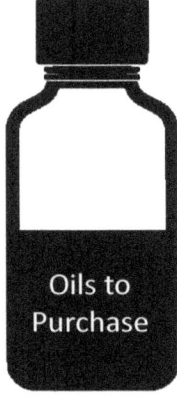

Oils to Purchase

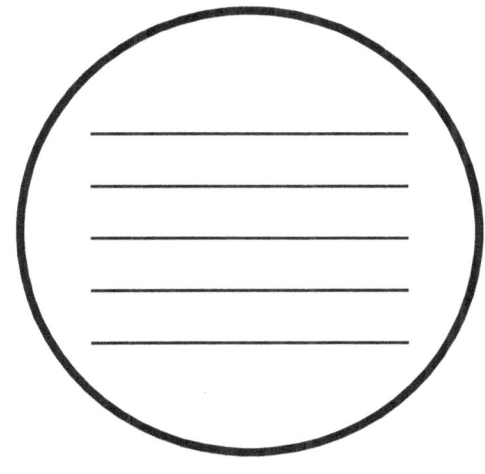

Daily Oil Usage Tracker

Date: _____

	S	M	T	W	T	F	S
Lavender							
Bergamot							
Eucalyptus							
Frankincense							
Lemon							

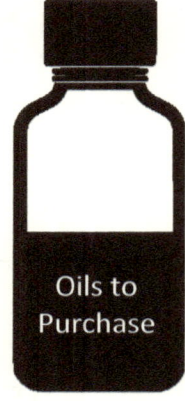

Oils to Purchase

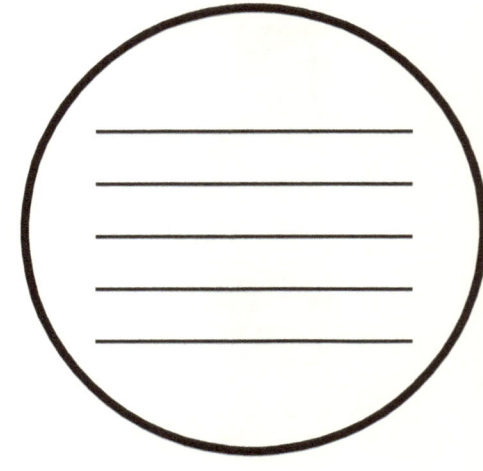

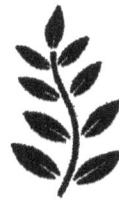

Daily Oil Usage Tracker

Date: _____

	S	M	T	W	T	F	S
Lavender							
Bergamot							
Eucalyptus							
Frankincense							
Lemon							

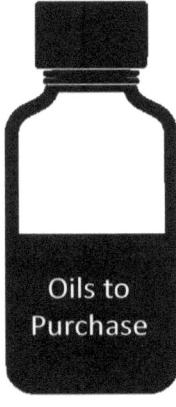

Oils to Purchase

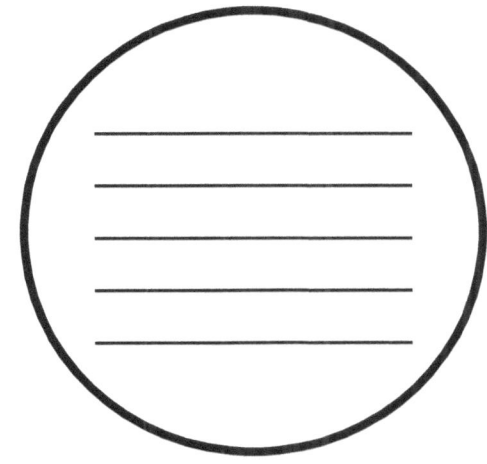

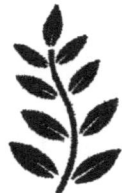

Daily Oil Usage Tracker

Date: _____

	S	M	T	W	T	F	S
Lavender							
Bergamot							
Eucalyptus							
Frankincense							
Lemon							

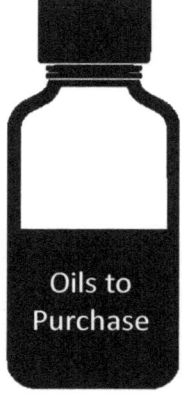

Oils to Purchase

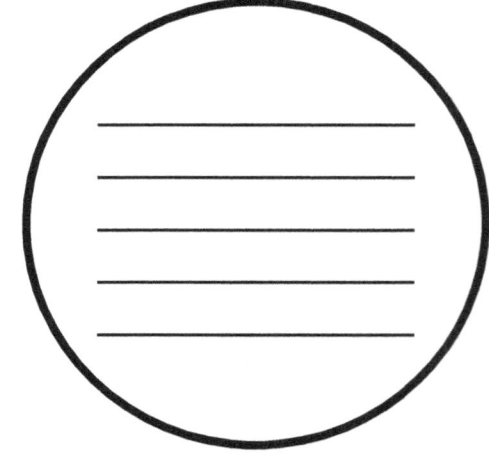

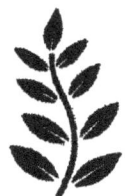

Daily Oil Usage Tracker

Date: _____

	S	M	T	W	T	F	S
Lavender							
Bergamot							
Eucalyptus							
Frankincense							
Lemon							

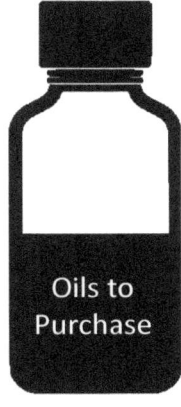

Oils to Purchase

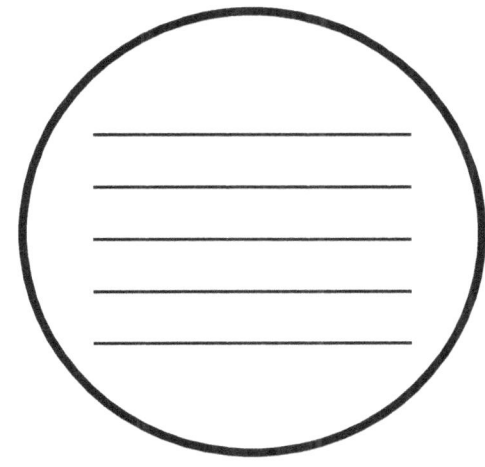

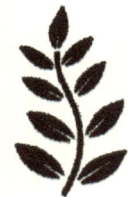

Daily Oil Usage Tracker

Date: _____

	S	M	T	W	T	F	S
Lavender							
Bergamot							
Eucalyptus							
Frankincense							
Lemon							

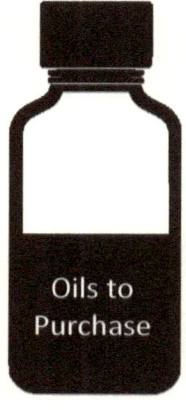

Oils to Purchase

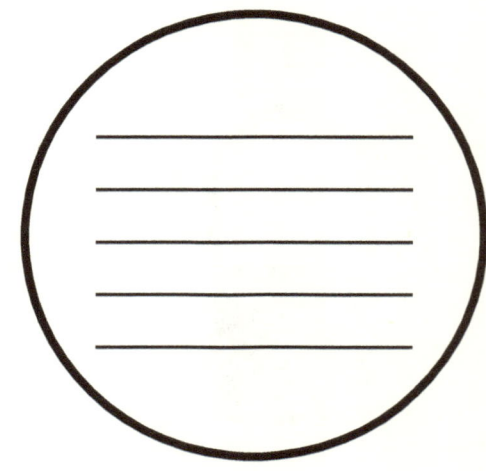

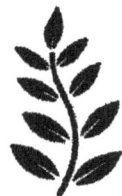

Daily Oil Usage Tracker

Date: _____

	S	M	T	W	T	F	S
Lavender							
Bergamot							
Eucalyptus							
Frankincense							
Lemon							

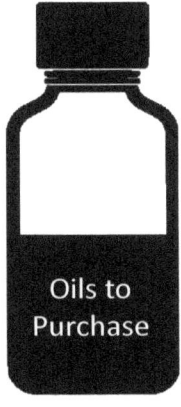

Oils to Purchase

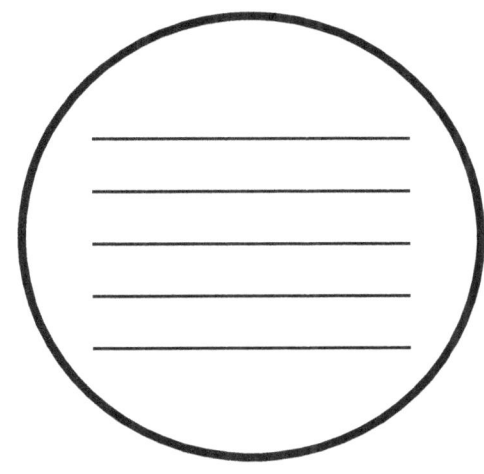

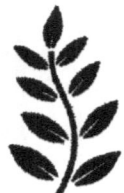

Daily Oil Usage Tracker

Date: _____

	S	M	T	W	T	F	S
Lavender							
Bergamot							
Eucalyptus							
Frankincense							
Lemon							

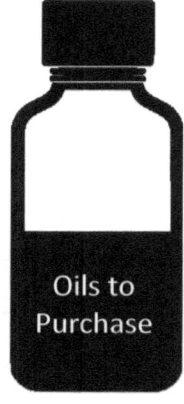

Oils to Purchase

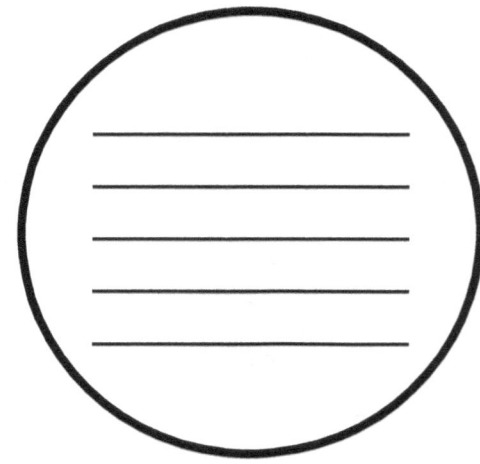

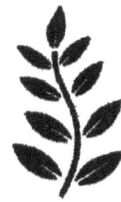

Daily Oil Usage Tracker

Date: _____

	S	M	T	W	T	F	S
Lavender							
Bergamot							
Eucalyptus							
Frankincense							
Lemon							

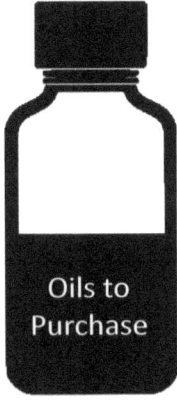

Oils to Purchase

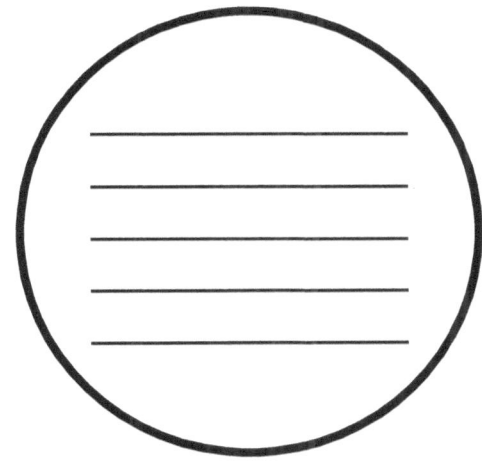

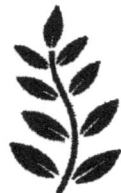

Daily Oil Usage Tracker

Date: _____

	S	M	T	W	T	F	S
Lavender							
Bergamot							
Eucalyptus							
Frankincense							
Lemon							

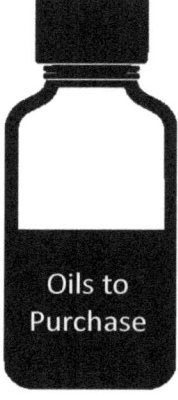

Oils to Purchase

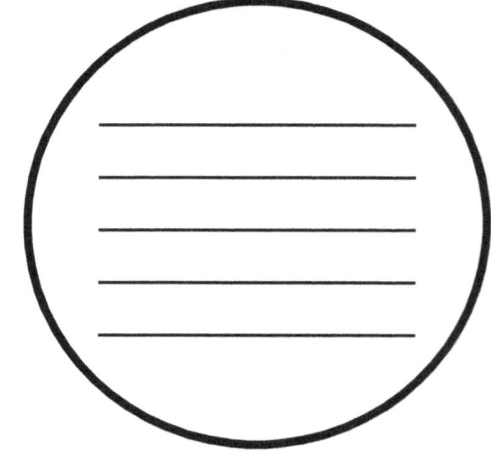

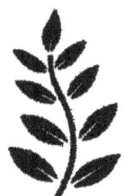

Daily Oil Usage Tracker

Date: _____

	S	M	T	W	T	F	S
Lavender							
Bergamot							
Eucalyptus							
Frankincense							
Lemon							

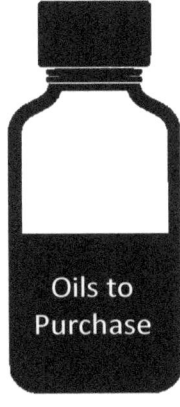

Oils to Purchase

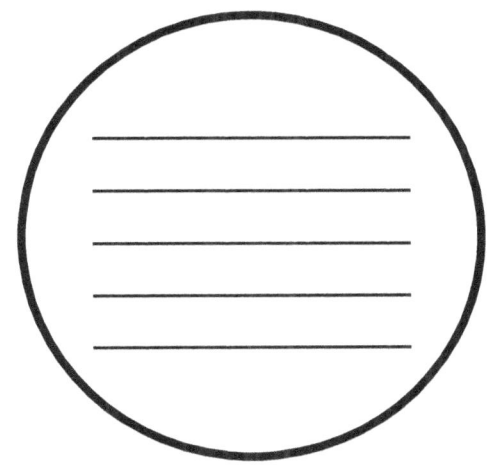

Daily Oil Usage Tracker

Date: _____

	S	M	T	W	T	F	S
Lavender							
Bergamot							
Eucalyptus							
Frankincense							
Lemon							

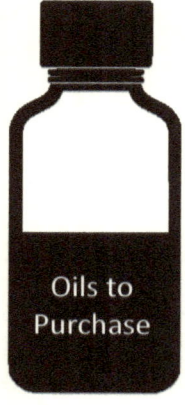

Oils to Purchase

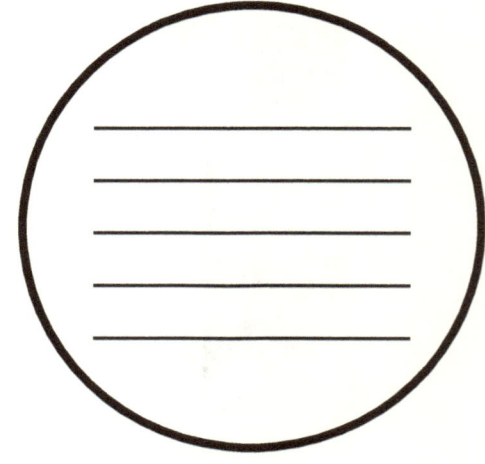

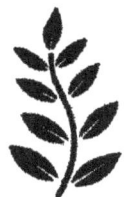

Daily Oil Usage Tracker

Date: _____

	S	M	T	W	T	F	S
Lavender							
Bergamot							
Eucalyptus							
Frankincense							
Lemon							

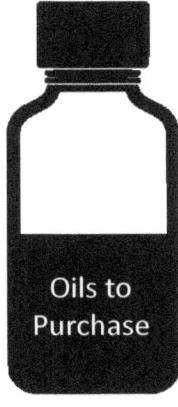

Oils to Purchase

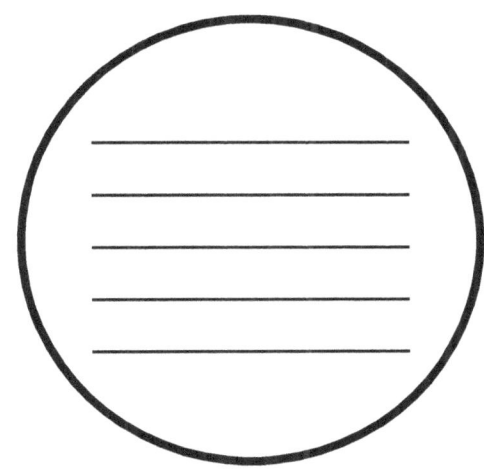

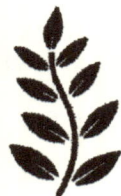

Daily Oil Usage Tracker

Date: _____

	S	M	T	W	T	F	S
Lavender							
Bergamot							
Eucalyptus							
Frankincense							
Lemon							

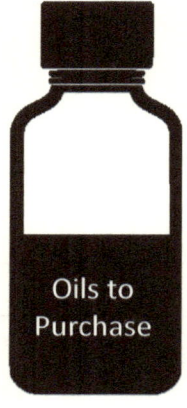

Oils to Purchase

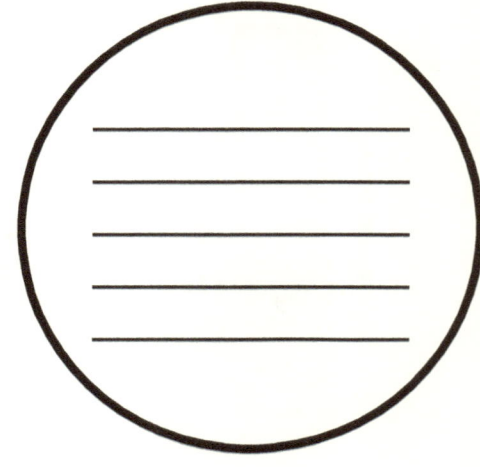

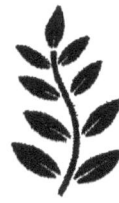

Daily Oil Usage Tracker

Date: _____

	S	M	T	W	T	F	S
Lavender							
Bergamot							
Eucalyptus							
Frankincense							
Lemon							

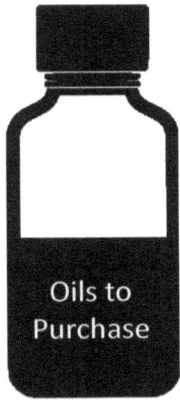

Oils to Purchase

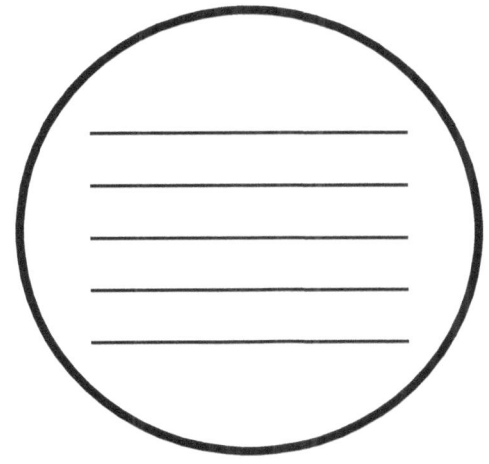

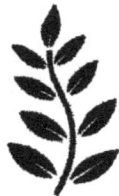

Daily Oil Usage Tracker

Date: _____

	S	M	T	W	T	F	S
Lavender							
Bergamot							
Eucalyptus							
Frankincense							
Lemon							

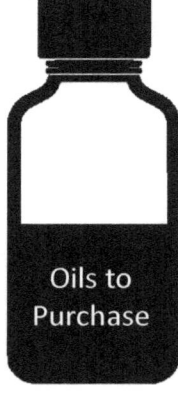

Oils to Purchase

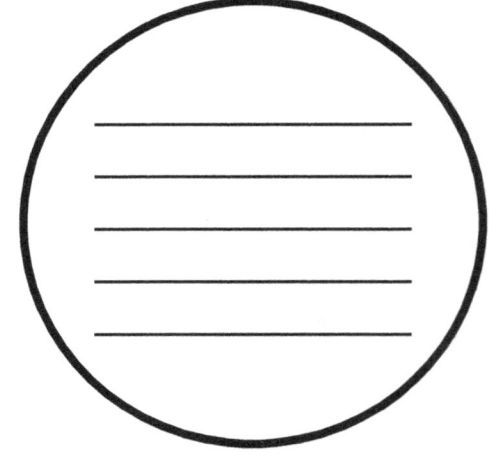

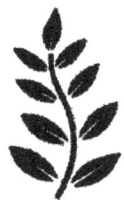

Daily Oil Usage Tracker

Date: _____

	S	M	T	W	T	F	S
Lavender							
Bergamot							
Eucalyptus							
Frankincense							
Lemon							

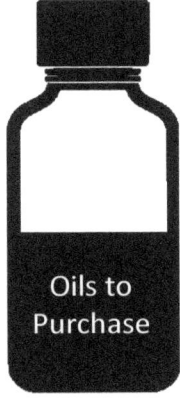

Oils to Purchase

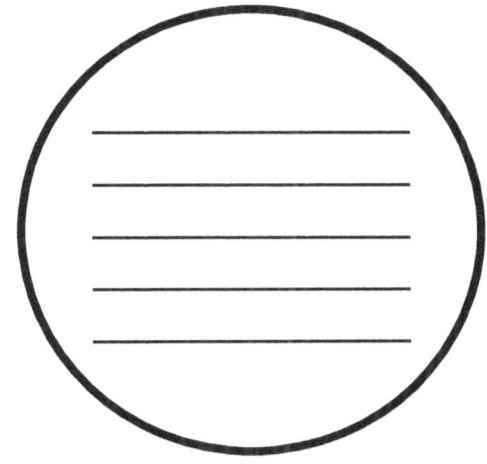

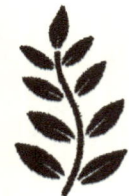

Daily Oil Usage Tracker

Date: _____

	S	M	T	W	T	F	S
Lavender							
Bergamot							
Eucalyptus							
Frankincense							
Lemon							

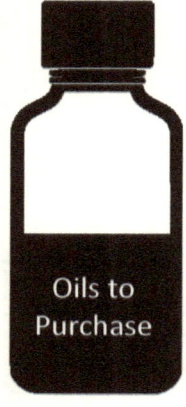

Oils to Purchase

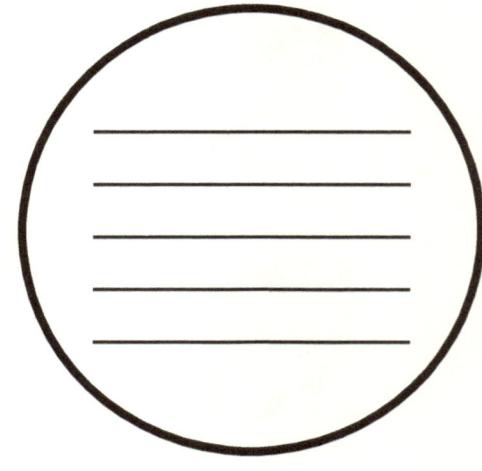

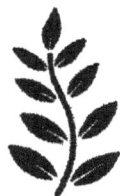

Daily Oil Usage Tracker

Date: _____

	S	M	T	W	T	F	S
Lavender							
Bergamot							
Eucalyptus							
Frankincense							
Lemon							

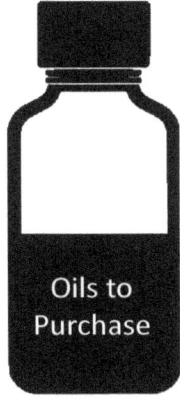

Oils to Purchase

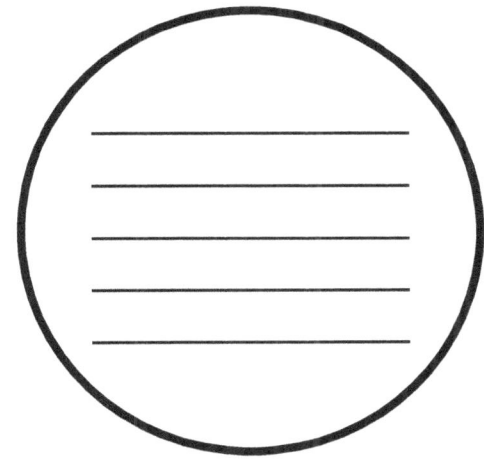

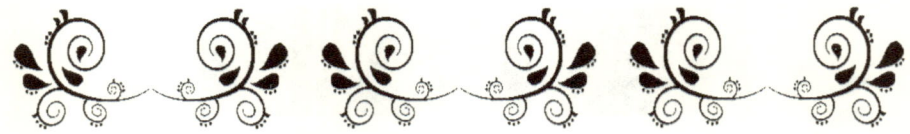

Wish List

Want	Buy From

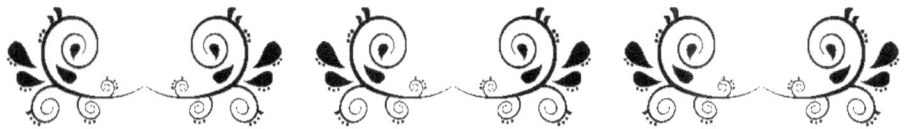

Wish List

Want	Buy From

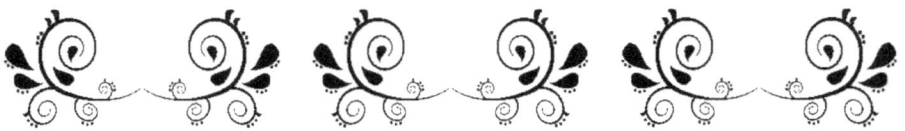

To Buy

Item	Buy From

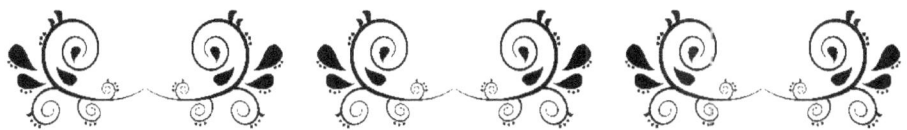

To Buy

Item	Buy From

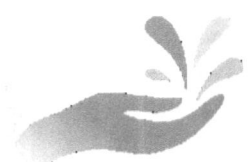

To Do

- [ ]
- [ ]
- [ ]
- [ ]
- [ ]
- [ ]
- [ ]
- [ ]
- [ ]
- [ ]
- [ ]
- [ ]
- [ ]
- [ ]
- [ ]
- [ ]
- [ ]
- [ ]
- [ ]

To Do

- [ ]
- [ ]
- [ ]
- [ ]
- [ ]
- [ ]
- [ ]
- [ ]
- [ ]
- [ ]
- [ ]
- [ ]
- [ ]
- [ ]
- [ ]
- [ ]
- [ ]
- [ ]
- [ ]

To Do

- ☐
- ☐
- ☐
- ☐
- ☐
- ☐
- ☐
- ☐
- ☐
- ☐
- ☐
- ☐
- ☐
- ☐
- ☐
- ☐
- ☐
- ☐
- ☐

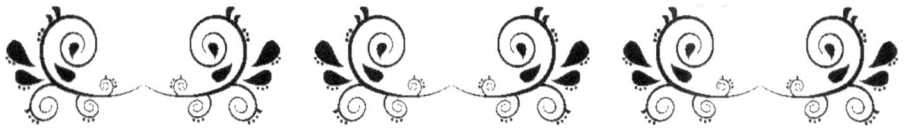

Perpetual Annual Planner

January	February	March	April

May	June	July	August

September	October	November	December

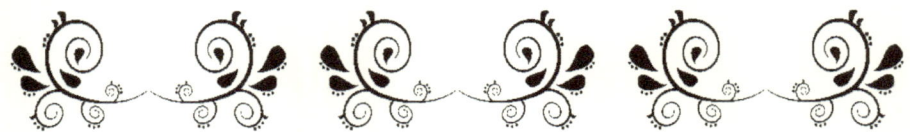

Herbal Book List

Book Title	Author

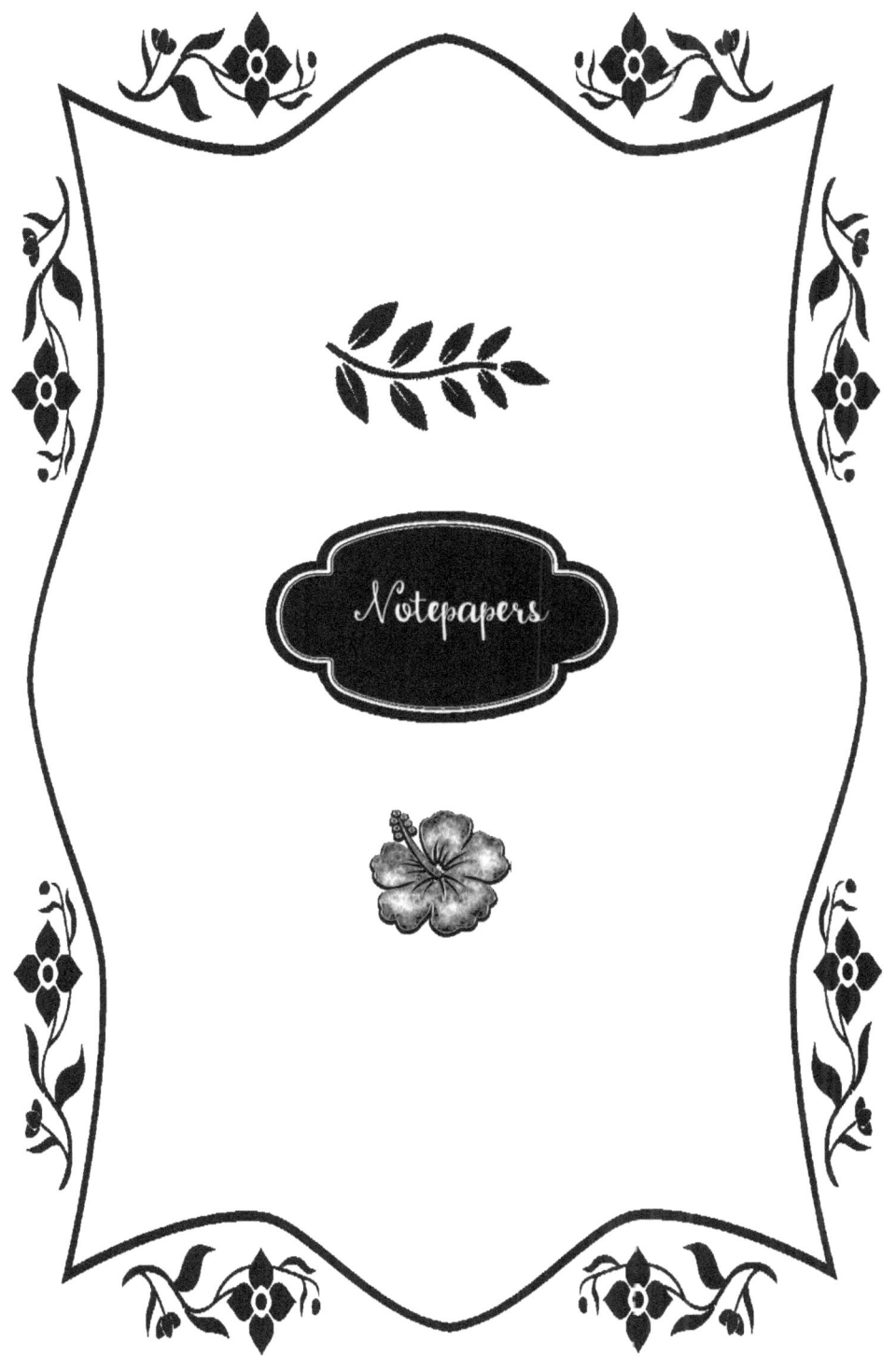

Notepapers

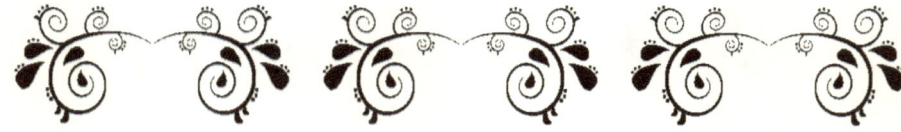

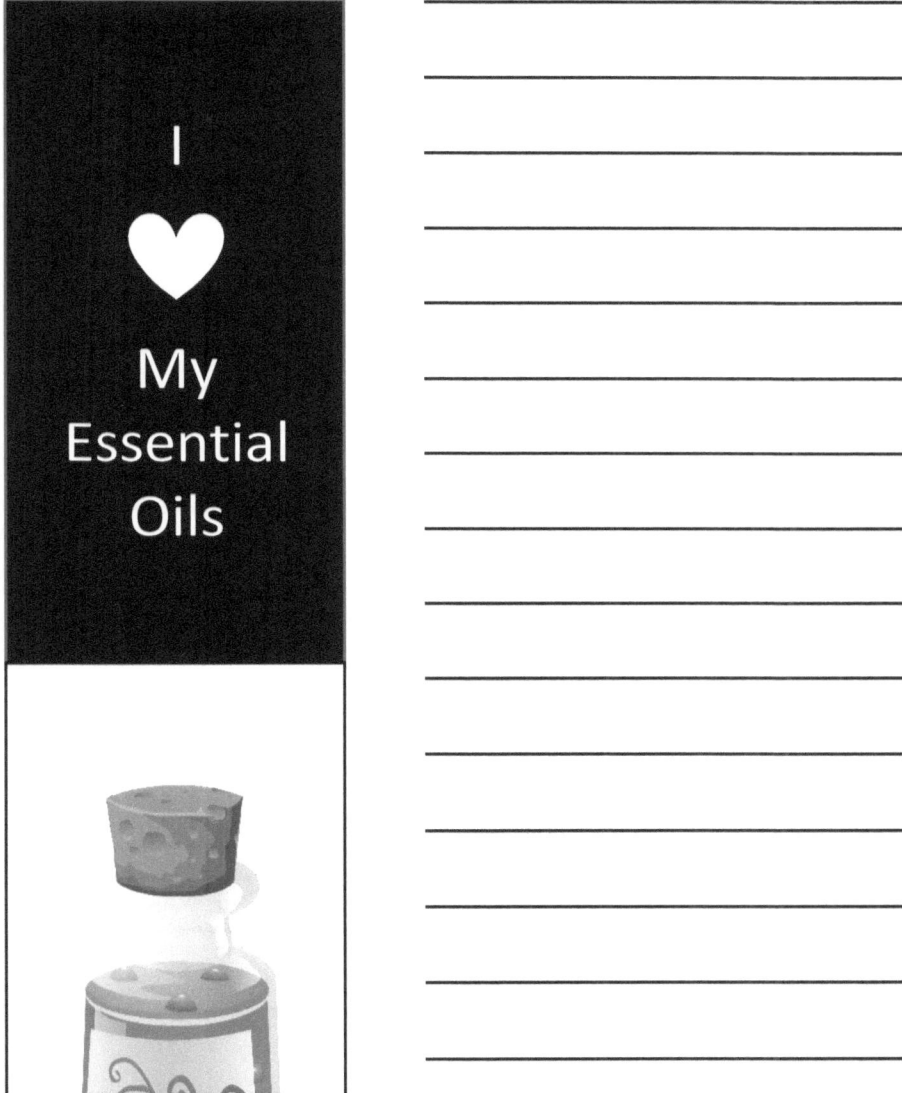

_____

_____

_____

_____

_____

_____

_____

_____

_____

_____

_____

_____

_____

_____

_____

_____

_____

_____

_____

_____

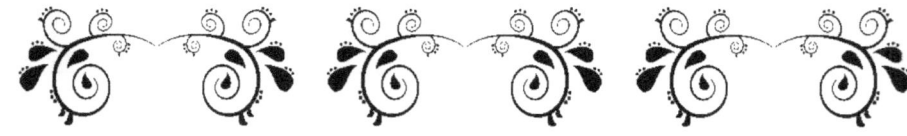

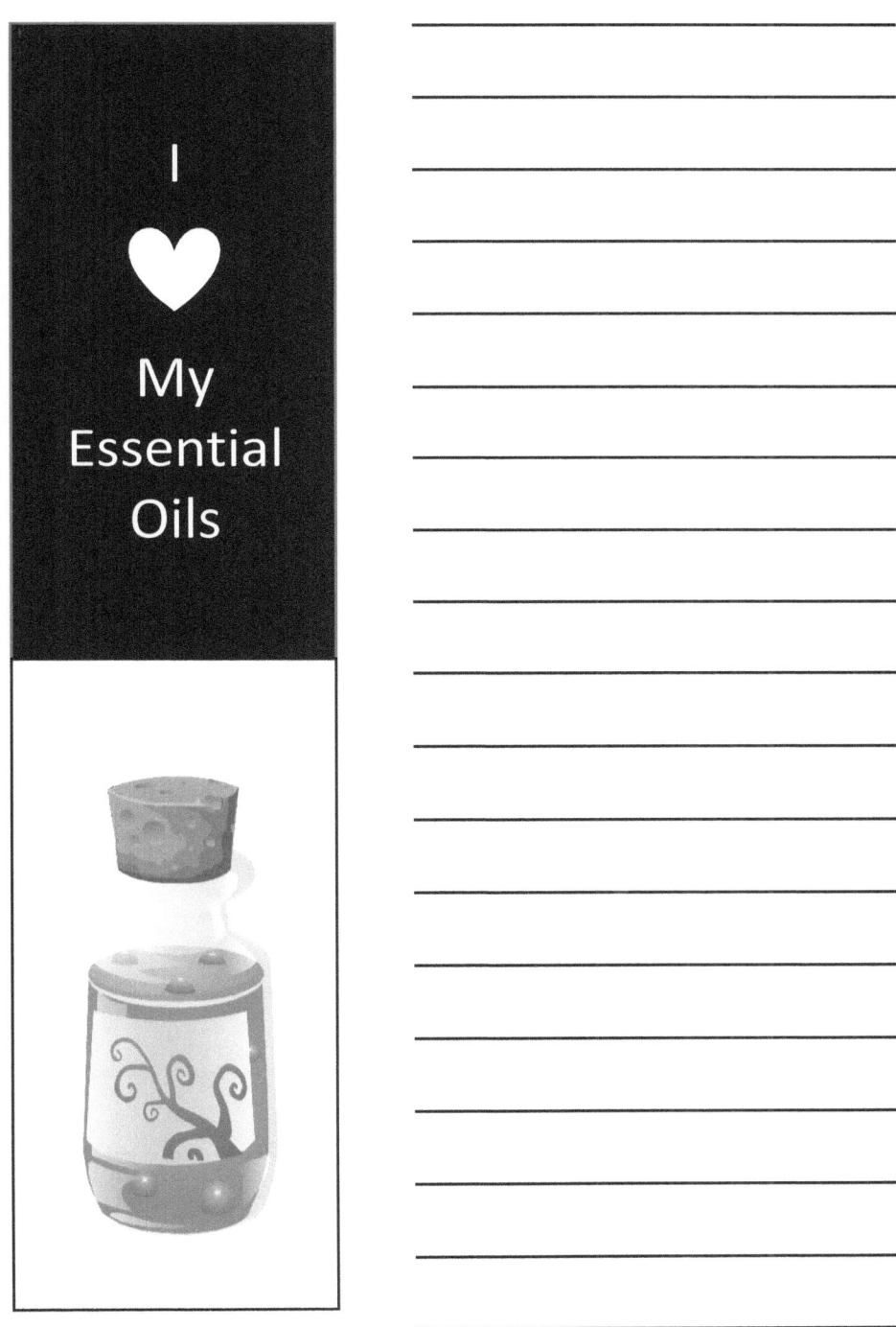

I ❤ My Essential Oils

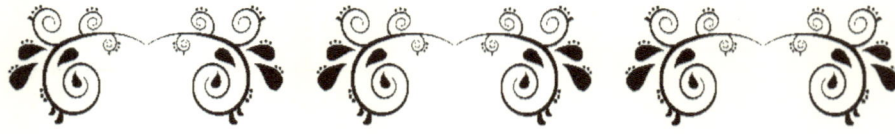

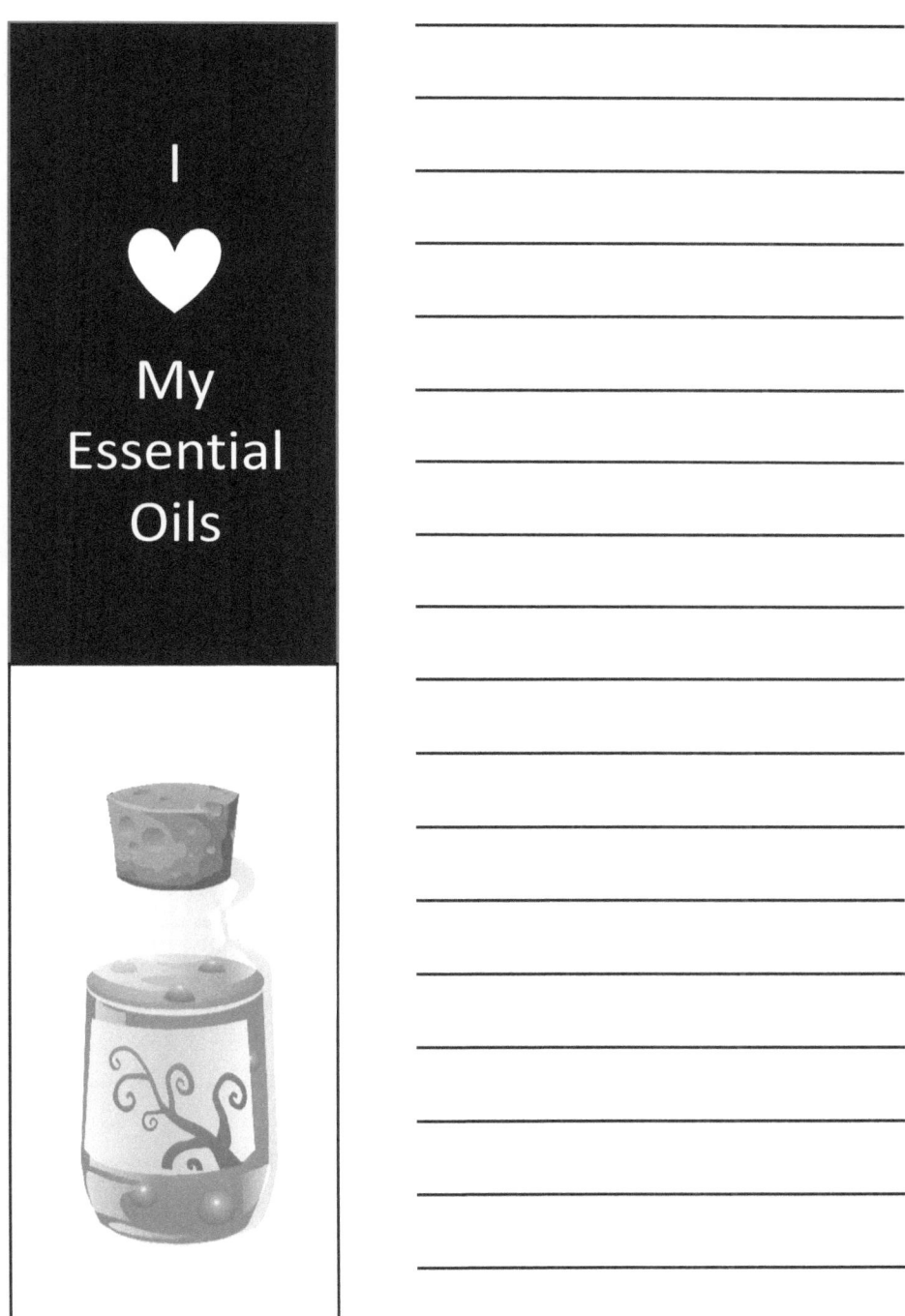

I ♥ My Essential Oils

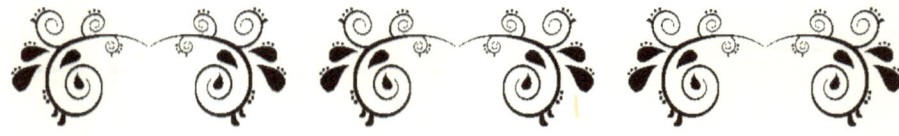

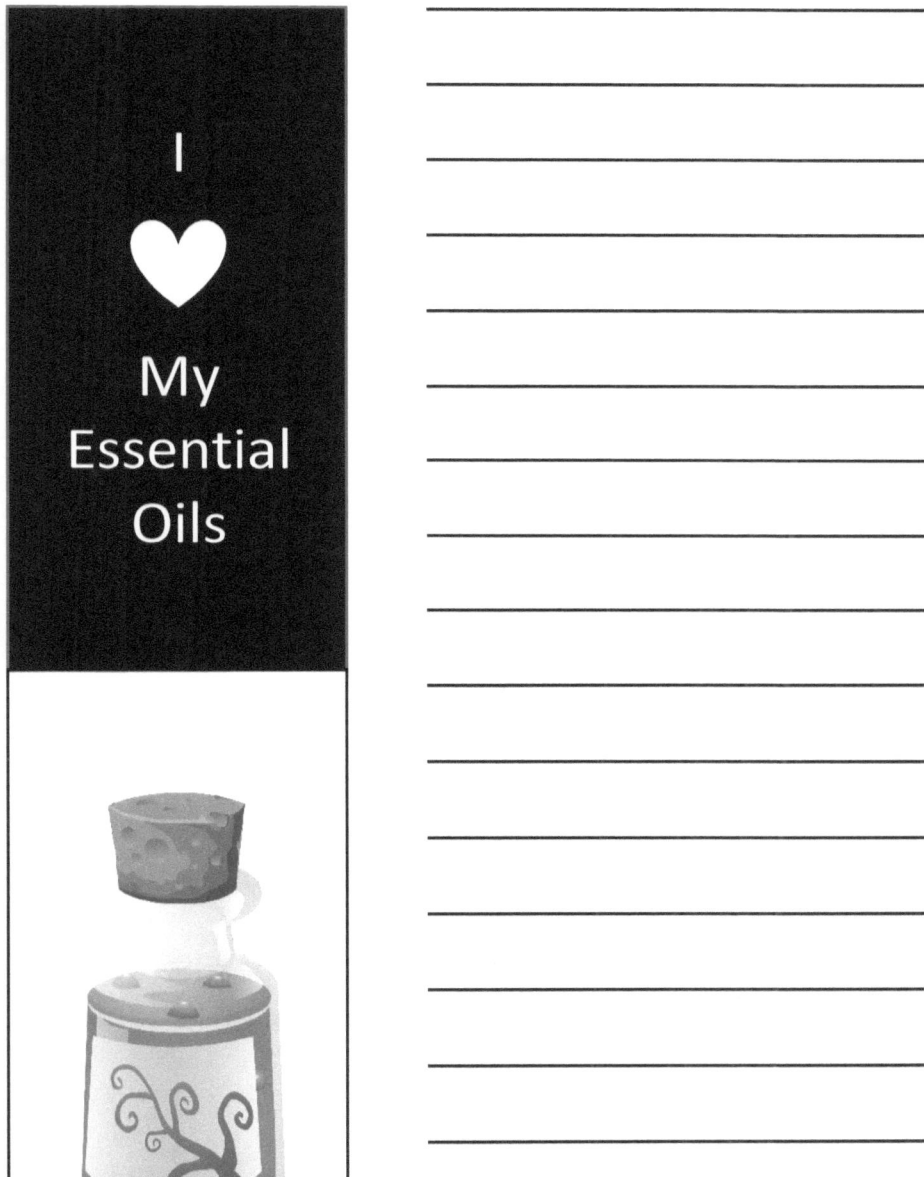

I

♥

My
Essential
Oils

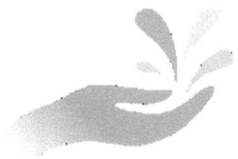

Thank you for your purchase of this Essential
Oils Planner and Tracker!

If you would like to learn about more resources
like this please check out
www.Reiki-Reconnections.com

and our Author Spotlight at:
http://www.lulu.com/spotlight/CarleneFord

The essential oils I use myself and highly
recommend can be found here:
http://www.mydoterra.com/reikireconnections

And do connect with me on Facebook here:
https://www.facebook.com/reikireconnections

- Carlene Ford

www.ingramcontent.com/pod-product-compliance
Lightning Source LLC
Chambersburg PA
CBHW020253290526
45784CB00003B/1234